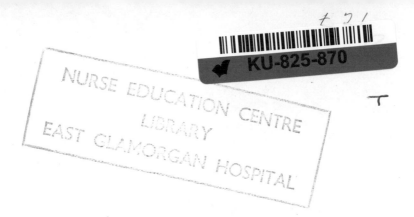

ON NURSING
Toward a new endowment

ON NURSING

Toward a new endowment

MARGRETTA M. STYLES

Dean, School of Nursing and
Associate Director of Nursing Service,
University of California, San Francisco

Illustrated

THE C. V. MOSBY COMPANY

ST. LOUIS · LONDON · TORONTO   1982

MOSBY

A TRADITION OF PUBLISHING EXCELLENCE

Editor: Pamela L. Swearingen
Assistant editor: Bess Arends
Manuscript editor: Judi Wolken
Design: Kay Kramer
Production: Judith Bamert

The C.V. Mosby Company
11830 Westline Industrial Drive, St. Louis, Missouri 63141

Library of Congress Cataloging in Publication Data

Styles, Margretta M.
  On nursing.

  Bibliography: p.
  Includes index.
  1. Nursing. 2. Nursing—Philosophy. I. Title.
RT82.S88   610.73'06'9   81-16980
ISBN 0-8016-4874-2   AACR2

To our professionhood—
Yours and mine.

CONTENTS

ON NURSING
Toward a new endowment

INTRODUCTION

1

THE INVITATION

I have never written a book before, so don't be surprised to find this volume a bit out of line with custom and etiquette. Since my major intent is to engage in personal conversation on intimate professional matters, the first person—I and we—and second person—you—will pop up frequently. This cannot be avoided, although it may make both of us uncomfortable at times.

It may also be disconcerting that I occasionally use terms of my own invention because they have special meanings for me that have not found adequate conveyance elsewhere. Then, too, I find some words in the "professional" constellation have become empty vessels from which the real significance has been drained through numerous verbal orgies. Moreover, it seems to me that, since language forms and conveys our thoughts and excites and motivates us, linguistic mutations are as important to extending thinking and feeling as genetic mutations are essential to improving biological makeup.

Still another way in which this writing strays from contemporary thought and practice is that it focuses intensely on nursing, not more widely on the health sciences, nor the helping professions, nor social institutions in general. Such absorption is not to pretend an isolation or independence but to acknowledge that our inner world—our professional identity—must be secure before we can turn outward with vigor and positive effect. This is true for all professions. *On Nursing: Toward a New Endowment* proposes and utilizes a process for securing the inner world of nursing and, indeed, that of other occupations that also have far to go in this crucial developmental task.

My ambitious endeavor in undertaking this book stems from the overpowering conviction that nursing has a great destiny but one that cannot be fulfilled until nurses—you and I and all of us—change what we are. For us to change what we are, we must change the way we think, the way we feel, and the way we act. Such transformations begin with discussions on a personal level in which we expose our thoughts and perceptions, in whatever stage of their gestation, to the light of our own self-appraisal and the scrutiny of others. Within these pages are my views on achieving our professionhood, offered in the trust that, mingled with yours, they will mature and prosper. In this way this work may serve as an instrument of socialization for us both as writer and reader.

Several features will appear in the attempt to foster a close, dynamic interaction between us. As far as construction is concerned, you will encounter throughout more of a natural ideational stream than a syntactical model. Too, the reflections proceed along a generative edge, not from a preconceived outline, and thus will be uneven in certainty, tone, and detail. In places spaces will be saved to encourage you to linger, deliberate, and perhaps even jot down your own thoughts, so that your personal copy becomes a record of your passage as well as mine. Also, surely, in socialization endeavors, the reality that most nurses are females deserves to be emphasized, rather than denied; therefore, the feminine gender will be used consistently where choices must be made.

––––––––

We should introduce ourselves. Who am I? A nurse. I have recently celebrated my twenty-fifth year in the profession. This milestone seems a good time to pause, to stand back, to contemplate, to stretch. Except for brief intervals as a hospital staff nurse and supervisor, I have been largely employed in nursing education—diploma, associate degree, baccalaureate, master's, and doctoral. I have been active, too, in support of a number of nursing causes and in the attempted resolution of issues. Credentialing and the structure and governance of the profession are foremost among these.

Who are you? Student, clinician, administrator, teacher, researcher, bureaucrat? Precareer, early career, midcareer, late career, postcareer, noncareer? What nation, race, or religion? Whatever our particular circumstances, we all need to seek, to shape, to savor our fate. This is our never-ending privilege and responsibility—the mark of humanness.

As this work unfolds, could we think of ourselves as looking into the mirror of nursing?

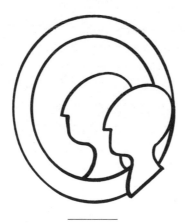

––––––––

The faces we see are our own. This particular writing is mine, but we are authors of the future of nursing together. Intoxicating, challenging, chilling, overwhelming, paralyzing, boring, tiresome—it may be one or all of these things, but the undeniable fact remains that our individual and collective destiny is, in large part, in our hands. To grasp this opportunity, we must have a strong sense of our professional selves.

This introduction holds out an invitation to search with me for a total view of nursing and for our personal meaning as nurses. Such a pilgrimage will take us first through the general field of professionalism as it has already been charted by others. Then, we will open up our own frontiers with the assertion of an ideology and directional model—a manifesto or social contract—for nursing; exploration of the nature of nursing and the conditions under which it is practiced; professional, academic, socialization, and governance models to enlarge our capacities and social legacy; and, most deeply, contemplation of those personal qualities that are passages to professionhood.

I must begin by explaining this last concept, that of professionhood.

2

PROFESSIONALISM AND PROFESSIONHOOD

An important distinction

A good point of departure in this journey to explore and secure the inner world of nursing is to consider the concepts of professionalism and professionhood. Why is it necessary to speak of *professionhood,* as well as professionalism? For that matter, why speak of professionhood at all? Doesn't professionalism cover what needs to be said and done? Is this a case of real conceptual difference or only semantic dalliance?

Checking with dictionaries or sociology references will be of no help. *Professionhood* does not appear in either. The suffix "-hood," connoting "individuals sharing a specified state or character" and used to create such evocative, almost spiritual, words as manhood, motherhood, brotherhood, and selfhood, is familiar to all of us. *Professionalism,* on the other hand, is almost too familiar. It has become unraveled around the edges in being pulled and tugged to encompass all activities engaged in for a livelihood, including sports, gambling, and prostitution. The expression, "he is a pro," is an example of this loose usage. However, applied with discretion, professionalism is still capable of a powerful import: namely, the conduct, aims, or qualities that characterize a profession. This meaning must be sharpened, of course, with a definition of profession. We shall get to that later.

Professionhood and *professionalism*—there is a critical, penetrating distinction to be made if we assume the license to do so.

Professionhood focuses on the *characteristics of the individual* as a member of a profession. Professionalism emphasizes the *composite character of the profession*. Professionalism, as the central concept, therefore, allows us to lose ourselves in the crowd; it permits the illusion of an "I-they" relationship; it even encourages a nonproductive or counter-productive range of responses from passivism, escapism, and blamism. On the other hand, professionhood, as the central concept, forces us to pay attention to our own image as the dominant figure in the mirror of nursing. It recognizes that

> **The professionalism of nursing will be achieved only through the professionhood of its members.**

Our efforts, yours and mine, to attain our professionhood as nurses and thus contribute to the professionalism of nursing, as well as to our own self-actualization, must be our major concern—therefore, this personal, voiceless dialogue, nurse to nurse. However, since our professionhood is shaped within the larger context of professionalism, a considerable understanding of the latter is required at the outset. The next section is intended to provide that foundation or to enlarge or reinforce an existing one.

FORETHOUGHT

You may find yourself approaching this overview of the literature on professionalism as you would a desert that you would rather not cross. But it would be better, if not entirely necessary, for our later discussions if you did not avoid the passage. It's rather short, as excursions into the literary culture of a particular field go, although admittedly some sources are quoted more extensively than necessary for a cursory understanding. These have been included in such detail because they are rich in insight and historical significance and valuable as references.

In large part, the authors cited are persons like ourselves who at other times and places were engaged in their individual searches for the meaning of their work. Their journeys preceded ours and will become part of our own. If the terrain seems arid, it is not because of the poverty of their thoughts, but because in scientific reporting we have been taught to squeeze the succulence of personality from our pens. Thus, too often, the paper presents the dehydrated self. To reconstitute the material, we readers must add the spices and juices of our own experiences, emotions, and opinions.

3

PROFESSIONALISM

As described

Professions and professionalism have been a major laboratory for sociologists for some time. Historians, educators, and members of many self-studying occupational groups have added their observations along the way. Organizing and reducing the prodigious literature that has ensued is a challenge, but one that is worthwhile, both for understanding nursing's past and present place in the social scheme and for plotting our future.

Professionologists (a neologism of the tongue-in-cheek variety) have approached the study of professions from a number of different angles. Some have defined; some have traced; some have described; some have critiqued. This review has been outlined accordingly, with segments on definitions, history, and characteristics in this chapter and critical appraisals in the next. First a description, then a critique. We can pick and choose from among all of these sources in developing our own perspective.

DEFINITIONS

Protocol and logic would dictate that the word "profession" be defined here without further delay, but this is no simple task, largely because of the plethora of experts and opinion and the range of facets encompassed in the definitions: for example, classification, purpose, activity, structure, values, tools, and training. Each facet relies on the others for additional validation, yet not all are embodied within a single, authoritative definition. It seems sufficient for our purposes to catch a glimpse of definitional changes over time, then to appropriate the composite of a centrist who has surveyed the field, and finally to mention those contemporaries who stray from classical interpretations.

The dictionary defines a profession as "a calling," specifically one that requires *specialized knowledge and often long and intensive academic preparation.* The use of the term "calling" is provocative in that it embraces the concept of divine influence with a heavy emphasis on inner, altruistic impulses. In this aspect, latter-day connotations bear a faint resemblance to the word as traced back to the Middle Ages and its derivation from "profess," meaning affirmation or avowal. Professions then were bound up with the faith they professed and with the values to be achieved by their services. "Thus, medicine professed health, law professed justice, education professed truth, the ministry professed salvation" (1: 146). With various social changes over the intervening centuries, other dimensions have been added to that of motivation and value orientation. A 1953 composite developed by educator Morris Cogan from a thorough study of the many definitions of the word serves well as a shortcut through myriad modern meanings:

> A profession is a vocation whose practice is founded upon an understanding of the theoretical structure of some department of learning or science [a discipline], and upon the abilities accompanying such understanding. This understanding

and these abilities are applied to the vital practical affairs of man. The practices of the profession are modified by knowledge of a generalized nature and by the accumulated wisdom and experience of mankind, which serve to correct the errors of specialism. The profession, serving the vital needs of man, considers its first ethical imperative to be altruistic service to the client. (14:49)

A number of somewhat less orthodox definitions enliven the field. Both Strauss and Taylor have developed the concept of occupations as *work environments*, each with its own attendant properties (46; 47). Within this context, professions, as just one of several work environments, are seen to possess the characteristics of expertise, autonomy, commitment, and responsibility (46:8-9; 47:123-124). Becker, a sociologist, provides the cynical touch; he finds the term "profession" to be primarily a *symbol*. In his opinion, professions can only be defined as "those occupations which have been fortunate enough in the politics of today's work world to gain and maintain possession of that honorific title" (5:32-33).

Professionalism, although an equally ubiquitous term, takes on a more inferred than direct meaning, stemming from its origin in the varying concepts of profession. Vollmer and Mills have used the term to refer to "an *ideology* and associated activities that can be found in many and diverse occupational groups where members aspire to professional status" (48:viii). Within this context, *profession* is an ideal rather than a reality; it is "an abstract model of occupational organization" (48:vii). Nor is the term *professionalization* very often explicitly defined, even though it is frequently used in association with profession. Usually, it refers to the *process* by which occupations and individuals modify their characteristics and move toward professional status. Vollmer and

Mills comment on the relationship between the two words: "Many occupational groups that express the ideology of professionalism in reality may not be very advanced in regard to professionalization" (48:viii). In the case of individuals, the word *socialization* (or acculturation), meaning the acquisition of the values, norms, and symbols of a group, is often applied.

These selected illustrations point out in abridged fashion the disparate approaches to defining professions and professionalism. They also reinforce the necessity for us to try to do so for ourselves.

HISTORY

At least three historical notes on professions and professionalism should be sounded because of their particular significance to our later deliberations on the development of nursing as a profession.

Professionalization and civilization

First, *professions in the modern sense have flourished only in highly industrial and urban societies.* The strength of the professionalization movement in the United States supports such a generalization, and an international survey should disclose its validity in predicting and describing the degree of professionalization of occupations in other nations as well.

The urbanization that was necessary for and intensified by industrialization brought together sufficient numbers of people to create the possibility of a livelihood for professional persons. For example, the complications of business that came with "manufactories" required accountants, and the advances of science and the wealth developed by commerce produced conditions for the development of engineering. Reader, in his book *Professional Men*, states: "The professions as we know them are very much a Victorian creation, brought into being to serve the needs of an industrial society" (36:2). The ancestry of the modern "old professions"—medicine, law, the clergy—can ultimately be traced to the basic needs for health, social order, and understanding. In the West for a period during the Middle Ages, the church played a major role in all three functions, as well as providing the education necessary to perpetuate them. With gradual differentiation, law, then medicine, and eventually education became secularized, a process that was substantially completed by the end of the sixteenth century (11:289-291). During the nineteenth century, the church-university lineage was joined with the guild line of surgeons and apothecaries, the common lawyers, and notaries to provide the antecedents of the modern professions (36:2).

The term "profession" conveyed a different meaning in the 1800s than it now does. In view of the position of medicine today, it is scarcely conceivable that as late as the 1870s medical degrees were granted for four months of study for each of two years (30:130) or that in 1910 Abraham Flexner found that many medical students were not even high school graduates. Flexner's report revealed that the proliferation of poorly trained physicians was such that, in many communities, physicians were unable to practice medicine as a sole means of livelihood (17:23-38).

The themes of change and steady evolution to be discussed throughout this chapter run through all the writings that consider the professionalization process. The dynamism is most vividly stressed by Anselm Strauss, who advocates that "professions be regarded less as rather stable communities of colleagues and more as temporary resting places within a historical stream of events—at which resting places men can be observed loosely organized under common title for certain common causes" (45:77).

Professions and universities

As a second major historical reference, it must be noted that professions and universities have enjoyed a significant relationship. In addition to spawning the "old professions," institutions of higher learning have played key roles in the development of emerging professions. Wilensky lists the establishment of a university connection as a stage in the natural history of professions in the United States (49:142-144). The diffuse structure of higher education in this country afforded entree to evolving professions far more generously than did the British system or the Continental system, which developed technical schools instead (34:46).

Insofar as universities are established for the purposes of discovering and transmitting knowledge and socializing students, and professions are the instruments whereby this special knowledge and competence are put to socially responsible uses, this alliance between professions and universities would seem to be a natural one. As viewed by Parsons, the core of the professional system lies, in part, in the "institutionalization of the intellectual disciplines in the societal structure" in the university (35:537). Nevertheless, internal tensions, common to all professions that have both science and practice components, have developed (26:2). The effect of this profession-university union on the value system and basic orientation of the profession and on the kinship between the academic professional and the practicing professional is a matter for serious consideration and often deep concern.

Professions and clients

A third key point from a historical perspective is that, traditionally, professionalism is thought of as rooted in two-party arrangements between the professional and the client. In the original sense, the professional is, in effect, an independent entrepreneur free to negotiate the terms of this relationship. Two of the more well-established professions, medicine and law, originated and have thrived within such a system in which controls, accountability, and fees are direct and clearcut. One sociologist has described early professionals as "guardians of the *laissez-faire* faith" (47:120).

New professions, such as accounting and engineering, have been practiced both independently and in organizations. Yet others, such as nursing and social work, are intricately bound up with the organizations that grew or changed with them.

Today, professions are predominantly practiced in organizational settings. Moore, quoting the 1960 U.S. census report, says that "over four-fifths (about 82 percent) of all male 'professional, technical, and kindred' workers in the United States were salaried" (34:187-188).

A host of factors influences the outcome of the mixing of professions and organizations, not the least of which are the combinations of employee role and organization characteristics. Schein (43) and others have identified the following as important variables in this relationship:

1. The *proportion* of the professional's effort engaged by the organization, ranging from a minor percentage to that of a major propor-

tion, with private practice as a supplement to primarily institutional practice

2. The *relationship* of the professional to the organization, including professionals who are partners in group practice, service contract employees, salaried employees, and ministrators within organizational hierarchies

3. The primary *product* of the organization, running the gamut from health services to corkscrews

As professions and organizations have interacted and evolved together in increasingly complex ways, client identification, which is a basic necessity for ethical and autonomous practice, has become more difficult. Multiple client systems, made up of primary-secondary-tertiary and immediate-intermediate-ultimate clients, develop. An occupational health nurse may view the workers, the industry, or the wider public as clients. The hospital nurse deals with patients, management, and third-party payers as clients. The faculty member, whose complicated, multitiered client field includes the student, the university, the health care agency for clinical practice, and the patient, may be in the most ambiguous situation of all.

The dilemma of client identification thus touches on a number of aspects of professionalism. As occupations attempt to develop along professional lines within an organizational-employer context—in which bureaucratic structures and individuals with different and often conflicting values are interposed between the two traditional principles in the professional compact—the bases for legitimate control and accountability are blurred and tensions are created. Control by professional peers versus control by organizational superiors becomes a critical issue with which institutional governance models must deal.

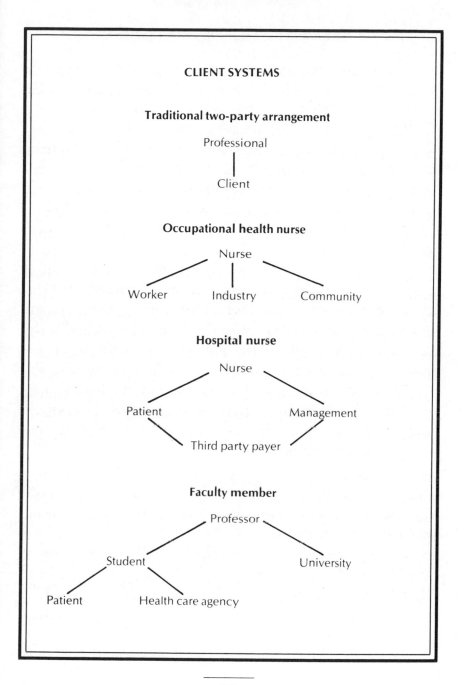

CHARACTERISTICS OF PROFESSIONS

The literature is amazingly repetitious with attempts to define professions and professionalism by their distinguishing characteristics. This recital of hallmarks has been such a popular approach to differentiating professions from other occupations that it is possible to compile a catalog of such lists. We shall be partially spared its complete contents. The following have been selected to convey the full flavor of the field by reflecting repeated emphases, as well as the more idiosyncratic views. Skimming them brings out both the sameness and the occasional eccentricity.

One of the first and still highly venerated formulations of criteria for professionalism was developed by Abraham Flexner, an educator best known for his 1910 study that led to the reformation of medical education and, not coincidentally, the elevation of the status of the physician. In 1915, when addressing a conference of social workers, he responded to the title question, "Is Social Work a Profession?" by listing characteristics that he deduced from observation of "professions universally admitted to be such—law, medicine, and preaching." His criteria, paraphrased, were:

1. Activities involved are primarily *intellectual*. Manual work or use of tools is not excluded, but the essence of the activity is intelligent problem-solving. This results in a large and personal responsibility for the judgment that is exercised.
2. Activities require use of knowledge that is not generally accessible. Laboratories and seminars provide new ideas and information which keep professions from degenerating into routine. This criterion is described as their *learned* character.
3. Activities have a definite, *practical* and concrete purpose. They are not merely academic and theoretic.
4. The *technique* employed *can be communicated* in an orderly way.

Members of a profession are in substantial agreement about what needs to be taught.

5. Members of a profession form a *brotherhood*. The social and personal lives of professionals and their families organize around the nucleus.

6. Members of professions are *devoted to the larger good*, not just to pecuniary interest. (18)

Carr-Saunders and Wilson, surveying the British scene some fifteen years after Flexner, identified a complex of characteristics for the term "profession," again using law and medicine as sources for derivation:

> The practitioners, by virtue of prolonged and specialized intellectual training, have acquired a technique which enables them to render a *specialized service* to the community. This service they perform for a *fixed remuneration* whether by way of fee or salary. They develop a *sense of responsibility* for the technique which they manifest in their concern for the competence and honor of the practitioners as a whole—a concern which is sometimes shared with the State. They build up *associations*, upon which they erect, with or without the co-operation of the State, machinery for imposing *tests of competence* and enforcing the observance of certain *standards of conduct*. Material considerations of income and status are not neglected, but the distinguishing and overruling characteristic is the possession of a *technique* [emphasis added]. (11:284)

Treatments by latter-day entrants into the field of professionology have been relatively consistent overall, with some variation on the same themes. In 1957, Greenwood, a social worker, listed the following "Attributes of a Profession," which I have summarized:

Systematic body of theory. This entails intellectual preparation as opposed to mere apprenticeship; theory construction via systematic research; a critical, rational approach to formulation in the field; division of labor between theory-oriented and practice-oriented branches; and extension of the length of training. Theory may be accompanied by a high degree of skill, as in the case of a surgeon, but skill, in and of itself, is not a distinguishing characteristic.

Professional authority. Clients, as compared to customers, have no choice but to accede to professional judgment inasmuch as they lack the background to diagnose their own needs or to decide which of several ways they might best be met. Clients are likewise unable to evaluate the quality of the service they receive. It is this characteristic that leads to the rarity of advertising among professionals. "If a profession were to advertise, it would, in effect, impute to the potential client the discriminating capacity to select from competing forms of service." (24:48)

This position on professional authority is particularly interesting in light of current emphases on patient education, self-help, and informed consent and also in light of recent Federal Trade Commission judgments that prohibitions against advertising are unnecessarily restrictive. But to proceed with the remaining professional attributes according to Greenwood . . . :

Community sanction. A profession tries to get community concurrence, formal or informal, with its claims to authority in a certain area. This takes the form of control of training centers (accreditation), of title, of license, and of judgment concerning professional standards.

Ethical code. Consisting of both formal and informal aspects, this balances the potentially dangerous monopoly granted by community sanction. Relationships to colleagues are usually cooperative, egalitarian, and supportive; toward clients, service of uniformly high quality is rendered without respect to compensation, client personal characteristics, or self-interest. Professional associations exercise formal discipline; colleagues exert a more informal pressure toward compliance with standards.

Professional culture. There is a network of formal and informal groups which, by their interrelationships, form a sub-culture. Although this occurs in nonprofessional occupations, the nature of the culture—its values, norms, and symbols—is different among professions and from one profession to another. A part of the training of the neophyte involves acculturation to a particular occupational group. (24)

In 1960, Goode, a sociologist, in the context of dealing with the territorial struggles among the social sciences, identified two characteristics as essential to professionalism: "a prolonged specialized training in a body of abstract knowledge, and a collectivity or service orientation," and an additional ten characteristics that are derivatives of that core:

1. The profession determines its own standards of education and training.
2. The student professional goes through a more far-reaching adult socialization experience than the learner in other occupations.
3. Professional practice is often legally recognized by some form of licensure.
4. Licensing and admission boards are manned by members of the profession.
5. Most legislation concerned with the profession is shaped by that profession.
6. The occupation gains in income, power, and prestige ranking, and can demand higher caliber students.
7. The practitioner is relatively free of lay evaluation and control.
8. The norms of practice enforced by the profession are more stringent than legal controls.
9. Members are more strongly identified and affiliated with the profession than are members of other occupations with theirs.
10. The profession is more likely to be a terminal occupation. Members do not care to leave it, and a higher pro-

portion assert that if they had it to do over again, they would again choose that type of work. (22:903)

As mentioned earlier, Taylor, following George Strauss, speaks of professions as a type of occupational environment, characterized by *expertise, autonomy, commitment,* and *responsibility.* Taylor amplifies:

> In the case of *expertise* it is asserted that the professional environment is one in which an advanced body of specialized knowledge and skills are required. These are usually obtained through long and demanding training, most often academic in nature. In maintaining the expertise of practitioners, occupational structures are established for training. In addition, norms for inclusion or exclusion of membership are also established.
>
> The *dimension of autonomy* in the professional environment is manifested in occupational structures which demand that practitioners be free to make their own decisions. In this way the professionals are set apart from lay restrictions. It is particularly at this point that conflict between the environment of professionalization and that of bureaucracy and unionization occur.
>
> The *dimension of commitment* in the professional environment often leads to the characterization of altruism as contrasted with individual aggrandizement. . . . In short, getting ahead in the environment of professionalism is as much measured by obtaining the esteem of one's colleagues as by advancement in one's place of employment or otherwise by economic measures. Commitment is to the occupational environment more than to what one can get out of it.
>
> The *professional dimension of responsibility* concerns control over practitioners, self-discipline, codes of ethics, and authority. The environment of professionalism is strongly built on boundary maintenances including the right to select, train, and control practitioners internally. . . . The authority of professionals may . . . be said to be subject-matter-specific. The authority of expertise is limited to a given

body of knowledge, and not ideally transferable to general situations [emphasis added]. (47:123-124)

Becker, again the iconoclast in the field, acknowledges the contents of the many lists of characteristics and concludes that the problem of characterization, as well as of definition, is the mixing of a technical, scientific, value-free use of the term "profession," with the popular, eulogistic, moral valuation usage. As mentioned in the discussion of definition, his solution is to treat the term "profession" as a symbol of something that actually does not exist but that people use in thinking about occupations. "It represents consensus in the society about what certain kinds of work groups *ought* to be like . . ." (5:38). In his opinion the symbol functions to legitimate claims to *autonomy*—the sole differentiating characteristic of a profession, according to Freidson and his followers (19:76).

Indeed, autonomy is viewed by many as the key value of professions. Dachelet and Sullivan, in writing about the role of the nurse practitioner, remind us that autonomy, as a central concept in professional practice, must be recognized as having two aspects: *job content* and *job context*. In their opinion, it is the former, relating to the technical or scientific aspect of the practice itself, rather than its organizational milieu, which is essential to professionalism (15). Would we agree? In fact, this belief may represent one of nursing's essential problems, deserving of fuller exploration in a later chapter.

We are often reminded that bound up with autonomy is the obligation of self-regulation or professional control. As stated by one author:

The question of control, after all, is the obverse of the question of autonomy, for autonomy is granted the profession with the understanding that it will itself, without outside interference, regulate or control the performance of its members. Just as autonomy is the test of professional status, so is self-regulation the test of professional autonomy. (19: 84)

Moore adds another qualifying note to the general discussion of autonomy by pointing out that there are both collective and individual aspects to this claim and that they may not always be compatible:

An occupation's claim to self-regulation, which is a kind of collective assertion of autonomy, has a doubtful relation to the individual autonomy of the professional. . . . Collective autonomy and individual autonomy may turn out to be inconsistent goals. Identification with peers may become subservience to peers, and that ends the effective sense of personal responsibility. (34:130)

An interesting approach, in differentiating between and among occupations, is that of Becker and Carper, who studied commitment to careers in various professional contexts. They identified four major elements of work identification: (1) occupational title and associated ideology, (2) commitment to task, (3) commitment to particular organizations or institutional positions, and (4) significance for one's position in the larger society (6:101). This is well worth giving a lot of thought to in our introspective and analytic moments and will undoubtedly surface in later discussions.

Some authorities focus their lists of characteristics specifically on the *nature of professional activity,* rather than more broadly on the traits of the professional collective. The National Labor Relations Act is perhaps an unexpected source of enlightenment in this regard. The Act defines professional employees as those engaged in work:

i. predominantly intellectual and varied in character as opposed to routine mental, manual, mechanical, or physical work;

ii. involving the consistent exercise of discretion and judgment in its performance;

iii. of such a character that the output produced or the result accomplished cannot be standardized in relation to a given period of time;

iv. requiring knowledge of an advanced type in a field of science or learning customarily acquired by a prolonged course of specialized intellectual instruction and study in an institution of higher learning or a hospital, as distinguished from a general academic education or from an apprenticeship or from training in the performance of routine mental, manual, or physical processes. (13:289)

The exclusion of standardization from professional work, which the third statement makes explicit, may jar nursing's sensitivities because of the protocols and standing orders that figure so prominently in our practice. Indeed, it has put us on the defensive. Darley, a nurse, in writing on the significance of the designation *profession* and on the nature of professional responsibilities, anchors his concept of profession to *judgment,* and emphasizes that "the kind of judgment which the professional person exercises cannot be *standardized* and, therefore, cannot be regulated effectively by any authority outside of the person" [emphasis added] (16:84).

An approach that has simultaneously brought into perspective some of the historical and contemporary elements of professionalism—that is, both the evolutionary process and the ideal characteristics—is that of identifying the *main themes of professionalization.* Hughes has recognized two sets of themes having to do with *detachment* and *change in status:*

An appropriate equilibrium [must be struck] between detachment and interest . . . between [the] universal and [the]

29

particular . . . between the theoretical and the practical . . . between the intellectuals and the professionalizers. *Detachment* . . . in the sense of having in a particular case no personal interest such as would influence one's actions or advice, while being deeply interested in all cases of the kind. . . . It leads to finding an intellectual base for the problems one handles, which, in turn, takes those problems out of their particular setting and makes them part of some more universal order.

Changes [in status] sought are more independence, more recognition, a higher place, a cleaner distinction between those in the profession and those outside, and a larger measure of autonomy in choosing colleagues and successors. One necessary validation of such changes of status in our society is introduction of study for the profession in question into the universities. (27:6-7)

Another alternative to developing checklists is the view that occupations lie somewhere on a *continuum of professionalization*, ranging from the completely unorganized occupational titles to the ideal reflected in the definitions and characteristics that have just been considered. The term "ideal" underscores the fact that, as Becker has contended, no occupation literally and consistently exhibits these characteristics all the time. But the term also conveys the motivating, powerful influence of the concept (5:33; 24:46,54; 48:vii). Sociologist Pavalko, in developing such a continuum model of professionalization, measures work groups along scales on eight criteria: *theory, relevance to basic social values, training or educational period, motivation, autonomy, sense of commitment, sense of community, and code of ethics* (8:2).

Wilensky has added to the continuum idea in elaborating his concept of the "natural history" of professions. He presents evidence supporting his belief that there has been a relatively consistent pattern in the appearance of the tangible characteristics—full-timeness, establishment of training programs, university affiliation, organization of professional associations, licensure laws, and so forth—of professions (49).

Having sampled, and perhaps overstuffed ourselves on the literature on definition, history, and characteristics of professions, professionalism, and professionals, let us move on to read what critics, both friendly and unfriendly, have had to say about the professionalism ideal and its consequences.

4

PROFESSIONALISM

As judged

Professionalism has received mixed reviews, and the professionalization movement and its study have had an abundance of critics, both among academicians and the general public. Some write objectively of trends and problems, others are frank advocates or biting detractors.

Barber's outline of problems, or question areas, in the sociology of professions serves well as a platform for these critical appraisals. He mentions first the difficulties associated with arriving at a *definition of professions*, which we have already discussed in Chapter 3. In addition, he has identified these five considerations:

Social sources of concern for the professions
The role of the university school
Emerging and marginal professions
Professional roles and organizational necessity
Professionals and politics (2)

I have appropriated these as headings for organizing various judgments rendered about *professionalism* and have added a final comment on *professionology* itself.

SOCIAL SOURCES OF CONCERN FOR THE PROFESSIONS

Barber identifies the interweaving of "moral, intellectual and practical" concerns as the basis for the interest in the professions of modern society (2:15). The mixed consequences of the profit motive in business turned attention in the early twentieth century to professional values as an alternative, causing some to see professionalization of business and related fields as a possible solution to social problems.

The advocates of professionalism are firm in the belief that the professional environment is the model for other occupations (47:115) and that, in general, the fundamental character of society will be improved by the enlargement of the scope for professional behavior (2:32). In advancing this position, Taylor has bluntly stated, "If the innovative, creative, high level practitionership of professionals could be obtained by alternate mechanisms there is little reason to believe that society would continue to pay the high price in prestige and remuneration currently awarded to professionals" (47:115). In effect, he has argued that the professional way is the only way for the public to gain these valued services. Other eulogists find professions a useful area for "defining central characteristic of modern society" and "as a vehicle for developing a general scheme of analytical variables that apply to all social action" (2:17).

Yet there are others who decidedly do not see professions as a panacea. Bernard Shaw may have spoken most sharply and most succinctly to the opposite view. "Every profession," he said, "is a conspiracy against the laity" (4:62). Roth has labeled professionalism as the decoy of sociologists, who, themselves, "up for grabs" as a profession, have been duped into becoming the "apologists for the professional ideology"

(42:6). He charges that the preoccupation with listing attributes and rating occupations has "deflected concern from the more crucial problems created by professionalization, such as the avoidance of accountability to the public, the manipulation of political power to promote monopoly control, and the restriction of services to create scarcities and increase costs" (42:18). With this one blow, Roth levels both the professionologists and the professions.

Professions have been denounced by those who see the professions' and professionals' insistence on autonomy and control as motivated by self-interest rather than community interest. Lack of accountability is a recurrent theme of public discontent. Hughes has pointed out that professionals "profess to know better than others. . . . they claim the exclusive right to practice." In addition, the professional "asks that he be trusted . . . [and] asks protection from any unfortunate consequences of his professional actions" (27:2-3).

Schein's summary of the concerns of society about the professions brings out explicit salient points and is well worth reading in its entirety:

> 1. The professions are so specialized that they have become unresponsive to certain classes of social problems that require an interdisciplinary or interprofessional point of view, e.g., the urban problem.
> 2. Educational programs in professional schools, early career paths, and formal or informal licensing procedures have become so rigid and standardized that many young professionals cannot do the kind of work they wish to do.
> 3. The norms for entry into the professions have become so rigid that certain classes of applicants such as older people, women, and career switchers are, in effect, discriminated against.
> 4. The norms of the professions and the growing base of basic and applied knowledge have become so convergent in

most professions that it is difficult for innovations to occur in any but the highly specialized content areas at the frontiers of the profession.

5. Professionals have become unresponsive to the needs of many classes of ultimate clients or users of the services, working instead for the organization that employs them.

6. Professional education is almost totally geared to producing autonomous specialists and provides neither training nor experience in how to work as a member of a team, how to collaborate with clients in identifying needs and possible solutions, and how to collaborate with other professionals on complex projects.

7. Professional education provides no training for those graduates who wish to work as members of and become managers of intra- or interprofessional project teams working on complex social problems.

8. Professional education generally underutilizes the applied behavioral sciences, especially in helping professionals to increase their self-insight, their ability to diagnose and manage client relationships and complex social problems, their ability to sort out the ethical and value issues inherent in their professional role, and their ability to continue to learn throughout their career. (43:59-60)

Continuing interest and distrust in the professions will be fueled by the fact that society itself is changing. Strong egalitarian sentiments are particularly sensitive to the allegations and appearance that professionalization is a *social class* issue (29; 31:264; 41). Barzun identifies Western impatience with authority and the "belief that anything long established is probably corrupt" as two general elements contributing to the animus (4). Further, the trust or "gullibility" of the public is undoubtedly eroded as the level of education of the public is raised (19:353-354; 20; 38). Mass education and mass communication undermine the knowledge monopolization that professions have held dear, resulting in greatly altered expert-client relationships and possibly in client revolt and the deprofessionalization of everyone (33). The evolution of professions collectively, together with social change, requires a revisionist attitude. In a concluding comment Barber leads us to expect more evidence of public concern and governmental action, as well as improved self-regulation by the professions. He has urged us to seek "solutions that pay their full respects to both egalitarianism, on the one hand, and specialized and powerful and useful knowledge, on the other" (3:615).

ROLE OF THE UNIVERSITY SCHOOL

The relationship of the professions to academia has created a second set of challenges to professionalism. Within the insulated academic environment, important intellectual, cultural, and ethical functions are carried out for the profession. Argyris and Schön summarize what they believe to be five central issues in professional education:

1. Whom does the profession serve?
2. Are professionals competent for practice in the current and future real worlds of diverse clients?
3. Does cumulative learning influence practitioners?
4. Is reform possible? [The authors point to schools as an unlikely source of change because of their separation from reality; practice sites as unlikely because of opposition from traditional practitioners; and both unlikely because expertise in reform is lacking.]
5. Can self-actualization occur? (1:140-146)

To these, Rosenstein, a professor of engineering, would add the question of values. He believes that professions have too enthusiastically embraced the value system of the pure sciences. In the pursuit of academic respectability, they have misdirected their principal orientation and energies from applied to basic research and, as a consequence, have not contributed as expected to the quality of life (39; 40). They have not fulfilled the promise, as stated by Parsons, to put this special knowledge and competence to "socially responsible uses" (35:536).

The university school is viewed by Parsons as the social institutional support for professions (35). In the same vein, Moore believes university-based professional schools have responsibility for setting high standards for both competent and ethical performance and for "sorting and authenticating" recruits to the field. Yet he believes both faculty and curriculum might be "graded on an awe-contempt scale," and he finds groups of examples for both ends of the scale (34:127-128).

Bucher and Stelling's longitudinal study of residents in psychiatry and internal medicine and graduate students in biochemistry was focused at this advanced level for the purpose of studying the final phases of lengthy socialization or acculturation to professions. They found that such students make their own choices as to which characteristics or practitioners to emulate, increasingly discounting suggestions of others in favor of their own evaluations of themselves and situations. Serious questions are thereby raised about the reality and quality of the internal controls that professions claim are developed through lengthy training. In the light of pervasive self-validation, the assumed effectiveness of colleague professional control should also be challenged (10: 270-275).

Many authors comment on intra-professional tensions between theory-oriented and practice-oriented individuals, deriving, some say, from the more basic incompatibility between the values of science and the values of professions (26:139-144). This sometimes assumes the form of strain between academic and practice branches of professions. Barber speaks of the stresses that are created as follows:

> The university professional is ever pressing, with increasing knowledge and higher moral standards, on the practicing professional who has to meet other pressures, sometimes . . . from nonprofessional organizations in which he works, but also from other cultural and social interests. (2:22)

EMERGING AND MARGINAL PROFESSIONALS

A third group of problems associated with professionalism surrounds the efforts of the outs to get in. A number of recurrent patterns become evident as occupations push to become professions and be recognized as such. The elite members of such occupations lead the movement for professionalization of the field, typically engaging in activities that highlight the characteristics of professional behavior. During this process of emergence, conflicts with elements inside and outside the occupational group occur.

Because there are rewards in the form of prestige and/or economic advantage for progression toward professionalization, occupations are sometimes seen to self-consciously measure themselves by the yardstick of generally accepted characteristics and attempt to meet them in mechanical fashion.

> Since symbols may hide the absence of reality, and the manipulation of symbols is often easier than the changing of actual organizations and behavior patterns, it is scarcely surprising that a considerable part of the observed behavior of organized technical occupations consists in the conscientious manipulation of symbols. (34:51)

As an example, Moore goes on to speak of the development of codes of ethics in this spirit of "checklisting":

Symbol and substance may get confused in social relationships, however. When established professions are observed to have certain common characteristics, those attributes may become definitional to all parties: to the accepted practitioners, to the laity, and to those occupational groups seeking to enhance their relative position (not to mention scholars analyzing the professions). Since a code of ethics is commonly taken as one criterion of professionalism, it is not surprising to observe aspiring groups ticking off the defining criteria, and formulating professional codes instrumentally. (34:118-119)

Along this same line, Hughes stops short of ascribing dual motives but notes that research is recognized by practitioners in emerging fields as accomplishing professional status for themselves, as well as development of new knowledge for service (28:67).

It has been suggested that the rapid growth in both proportion and absolute numbers of professionals from 1930 to 1960 may have had various consequences. "Continual growth has brought saturation, less quality, semi-professionals, and the echoes at least of deprofessionalization," according to Taylor (47:122). We in nursing with our burgeoning numbers and levels must pay special attention to this admonition. Both Wilensky (49) and Goode (23) doubt that professions in the precise sense will continue to proliferate indefinitely.

Resistance to the professionalization of aspiring occupations comes from both inside and outside the emerging group. As to external reluctance, Roberts, a nurse from Canada and Australia, attributes obstructionist attitudes to the established professions, who, cognizant of the finite professional rewards granted by society, oppose moves by other occupations toward professionalization. This is the motive she imputes to physicians who question why nurses need advanced knowledge and education (38).

On the other hand, we are all intimately and painfully aware of the disaffection with professionalization within the would-be professions themselves. Ritti, Ference, and Goldner have argued that what is suspect by the professional is not the beliefs, but "the organizational and institutional embodiment of these beliefs . . . the occupational myth rather than the belief system" (37:43). Stresses exist between the professional and the employing organization and "between the idealized and the day-to-day profession" (37:48).

As an example of this opposition within our profession, a group of writers, who identify themselves as the Boston Nurses Group, have aired their distrust in an article entitled "The False Promise: Professionalism in Nursing." They have stated that "professionalism not only does not serve our interests and those of our patients, but more often leaves us feeling unsatisfied, powerless, and isolated from other health care workers" (9:20).

PROFESSIONAL ROLES AND ORGANIZATIONAL NECESSITY

As a fourth area of concern, introduced earlier among the historical notes, professionalism is also considered a mixed blessing because of the difficulties involved in operating within a bureaucratic context. Not surprisingly, a confluence of professional, business, and intellectual interests is found in this problem area of professional and organizational interaction. Hughes says:

Most of the new professions, or would-be professions, are practised only in connection with an institution. Their story is thus that of the founding, proliferation or transformation of some category of institutions: schools, social agencies, hospitals, libraries, and many others. Whether the institution be new or whether it be an old one transformed, there is likely to be a struggle of the new profession with the other occupations involved (if there are any), and with the laymen who have some voice in the institution—a struggle for definition of the part of each in the functioning of the institution. (26:133)

There is consensus that the presence of professionals in organizations has modified in some measure the classical bureaucratic forms. The university is cited as an example of this interpenetration of the two forms. The need to preserve the freedom of the professional, a prerequisite for productivity, while at the same time giving another group authority to coordinate, is at the core of the problem (49:156). Barber has identified three accommodative mechanisms adopted to ease the strain that exists when professions clash with the organizations in which they are practiced: *differentiated role structures, differentiated authority structures,* and *differentiated reward structures* (2:26). These mechanisms provide ways to recognize in legitimate fashion the special expertise of the professional, yet maintain the integrity of the institutional structure. Under the best of accommodations, however, professional life is complicated inasmuch as the relationship to the client—be he person or corporation—is enmeshed in a web of other relationships (28:68).

Considerable attention has been given to the limits imposed by organizational context, especially those contexts in which organizations become the client. Under such circumstances professionals can lose autonomy, since the organization can find another engineer or lawyer or nurse if it does not like the behavior of incumbents. Consulting firms that locate professionals for business firms contribute to the phenomenon of dispensability. Increasingly, organizational clients hire one set of professionals to check on another. As corporate clients become more powerful, the professions become less clear about what standards and ethics should govern their relationships with them (43:29-31). The perspective necessary to provide effective professional service may be lost if the professional identifies too closely with the organizational client culture. Wilensky believes that organizations interfere less with technical expertise than with the service ideal, a more vulnerable characteristic (49:148).

The situation in which predominantly female professions find themselves is characteristically different from that of work groups whose members are predominantly male. The interaction of interrupted careers and geographical mobility with organizational setting puts such women's groups at a disadvantage in the organizational-professional negotiation process (44:246-247).

Organizations, whether academic or industrial, are not all bad, however. Of the practice institution, Kornhauser says:

> Students of the professions have tended to treat the need for functional autonomy of professions as the primary requirement; they see only the negative consequences of bureaucracy for professionalism. Thus they generally fail to analyze the profession's need for organizational resources and its contributions to the goals of organizations. . . .
> What we are suggesting is that *the tension between the autonomy and integration of professional groups, production groups, and other participants tends to summon a more effective structure than is attained where they are isolated from one another or where one absorbs the other.* (32:292-293)

Clark, describing the university, speaks in a similar vein:

In this situation, professional authority and bureaucratic authority are both necessary, for each performs an essential function: professional authority protects the exercise of the special expertise of the technologist, allowing his judgment to be pre-eminent in many matters. Bureaucratic authority functions to provide coordination of the work of the technologists with the other major elements of the firm. Bureaucratic direction is not capable of providing certain expert judgments; professional direction is not capable of providing the over-all coordination. (12:287-288)

Not only do organizations have some redeeming features, but it must also be recognized that private practice has some tyrannies and drawbacks that are overlooked by outsiders. The need to establish and maintain facilities, retain assistants, and manage a small business introduces constraints. Whether clients come by lay or colleague referral, the need to attract and satisfy clients further limits the unbounded autonomy usually attributed to private practice. Even professional judgment is influenced, since client perceptions of what they need and like affect referral and retention (5:42-43). Hughes describes this situation as paradoxical:

Here we are at a paradox of modern professional freedom. The effective freedom to choose one's special line of work, to have access to the appropriate clients and equipment, to engage in that converse with eager and competent colleagues which will sharpen one's knowledge and skill, to organize one's time and effort so as to gain that end, and even freedom from pressure to conform to the client's individual or collective customs and opinions seem, in many lines of work, to be much greater for those professionals who have employers and work inside complicated and even bureaucratic organizations than for those who, according to the traditional concept, are in independent practice. (28:69-70)

If the professional-institutional dynamic requires constant attention, how about that of the profession and the government? This leads to another problem area.

PROFESSIONALS AND POLITICS

The fifth and last set of challenges to professionalism to be discussed here relates to professionals and politics. In an era that has witnessed the increasing influence of experts on governmental policy (7), it is not surprising that this is an area meriting study. Professionals are increasingly retained as employees of government and are consulted for testimony in specialized areas. The difficulty in determining where expert knowledge ends and where the political and moral judgment begins creates problems for professionals and politicians alike (2:30). Professionals also engage in politics as organized pressure groups, particularly in relation to policies and funding that affect education, research, and other professional activities. Yet professions have not joined forces with one another in a major way to present a united front on issues of mutual concern.

In *Hidden Hierarchies*, Gilb thoroughly reviews professional associations, which she views as *private governments formed for the purpose of dealing with public governments.* Her examination of the internal politics, the frequently oligarchic forms of government, the disproportionate staff influence, and the specialized constituencies at once destroys romantic illusion and constructs a useful perspective. Another paradox!

> One of the paradoxes of American life is that when Americans talk about freedom for the individual, they generally band together into organizations to do it. Why does the

paradox exist—for example, in the professions? Freedom in a complex, interdependent economy comes *through* organizations. Without an organization to define and sustain his areas of freedom, the average individual professional would often not be able to be free. (21:53)

Schein, however, is less optimistic about the effectiveness of powerful professional organizations, observing that with increased power have come increased bureaucracy and decreased response to requests for support by members attempting to resist organizational pressures (43:48). Ah, nursing knows this well!

It is clear that critical appraisals about professionalism and professions are many and varied. Critics can be found on both sides of the issues, which range from self-interest versus community interest, the blending of professional and academic values, the behaviors of aspiring professions, professional and organizational interactions, and influence on government.

But how about professionology itself? As a final word, what can be said about the ways of conceptualizing occupations and of distinguishing the professions among them?

APPROACHES TO PROFESSIONOLOGY

In 1978 Klegon described the study of professions as being on the verge of transition. The taxonomic attempts at constructing lists, seen as too static and too difficult to apply because of differing and inconsistent terminology, are giving way to increased emphasis "on the factors affecting the ability of practitioners to organize themselves and manipulate the social position of their occupations" (31:259). Greater attention is being paid to the internal-external dynamics of profes-

---

sionalism, which involves "relating professional organization and control to other institutional forces and arrangements of power" (31:271). The sociology of work is shifting to this focus on sources of power and authority, subjects not easily amenable to checklisting. Terms such as organizational context and ecological processes are creeping into the professionology vocabulary as symbols of this new emphasis (25).

Thus it is apparent that the traditional view of professions, professionalism, and professionology—the entire sociology of work—is undergoing reevaluation and change.

5

PROFESSIONALISM

As summarized

Professions have grown in the context of urbanization and industrialization with the support, particularly in the United States, of the universities. Numerous lists of criteria for professions have been developed. These multiple variations in expression, format, and priority seldom stray from the universal themes of service commitment, ethical behavior, a particular expertise, a particular body of scientific knowledge, extensive university education, the spirit and form of collegiality, and autonomy in setting standards of education and practice.

Although the contributions of work groups commonly labeled as professions are generally acknowledged, tensions are abundant between:

- generalization and specialization
- academic and practice branches
- ideal and real
- false claims and legitimate bases
- professions and their work environments
- self-interest and community interest
- professions and governments

New approaches to the study and development of special work environments, such as professions, are being sought. Should nursing join in the search or adhere to the classical professionalization model? That should be our next discussion.

REFERENCE LIST FOR SECTION TWO

1. Argyris, C., & Schön, D.A. *Theory in practice: Increasing professional effectiveness.* San Francisco: Jossey-Bass Publishers, 1974.
2. Barber, B. Some problems in the sociology of the professions. In K.S. Lynn and the Eds. of Daedalus (Eds.), *The professions in America.* Boston: Houghton-Mifflin, 1965.
3. Barber, B. Control and responsibility in the powerful professions. *Political Science Quarterly,* 1978, *93*(4), 599-615.
4. Barzun, J. The professions under siege. *Harper's,* October 1978, pp. 61-68.
5. Becker, H.S. The nature of a profession. In N.B. Henry (Ed.), *Education for the professions.* Chicago: University of Chicago Press, 1962.
6. Becker, H.S., & Carper, J. Professional identification. In H.W. Vollmer & D.L. Mills (Eds.), *Professionalization.* Englewood Cliffs, N.J.: Prentice-Hall, 1966.
7. Benveniste, G. *The politics of expertise* (2nd ed.). San Francisco: Boyd and Fraser, 1977.
8. Bernhard, L.A., & Walsh, M. *Leadership: The key to the professionalization of nursing.* New York: McGraw-Hill, 1981.
9. Boston Nurses Group. The false promise: Professionalism in nursing. *Science For the People,* 1978, *10*(3), 20-34.
10. Bucher, R., & Stelling, J.G. *Becoming professional.* Beverly Hills, Calif.: Sage Publications, 1977.
11. Carr-Saunders, A.M., & Wilson, P.A. *The professions.* Oxford: Clarendon Press, 1933.
12. Clark, B. Organizational adaptation to professionals. In H.W. Vollmer & D.L. Mills (Eds.), *Professionalization.* Englewood Cliffs, N.J.: Prentice-Hall, 1966.
13. Cleland, V. The professional model. *American Journal of Nursing,* 1975, *75,* 288-292.
14. Cogan, M.L. Toward a definition of profession. *Harvard Educational Review,* 1953, *23*(33).
15. Dachelet, C.Z., & Sullivan, J.A. Autonomy in practice. *Nurse Practitioner,* 1979, *4*(2), 15-22.
16. Darley, W. The professions and professional people. *Nursing Forum,* 1961-1962, *1*(1), 83-89.
17. Flexner, A. *Medical education in the United States and Canada.* (A report to the Carnegie Foundation for the Advancement of Teaching). Boston: The Merrymount Press, 1910.
18. Flexner, A. Is social work a profession? *School and Society,* 1915, *1*(26), 901-911.

19. Freidson, E. *Profession of medicine: A study of the sociology of applied knowledge.* New York: Dodd, Mead, 1972.
20. Gartner, A. *The preparation of human service professionals.* New York: Human Sciences Press, 1976.
21. Gilb, C. *Hidden hierarchies: The professions and government.* New York: Harper & Row, 1966.
22. Goode, W.J. The profession: Reports and opinion. *American Sociological Review,* 1960, *25,* 902-914.
23. Goode, W.J. The theoretical limits of professionalization. In A. Etzioni (Ed.), *The semi-professions and their organization: Teachers, nurses, social workers.* New York: The Free Press, 1969.
24. Greenwood, E. Attributes of a profession. *Social Work,* 1957, *2*(4), 45-55.
25. Hall, R. The social construction of the professions. *Sociology of Work and Occupations,* 1979, *6*(1), 124-126.
26. Hughes, E.C. *Men and their work.* Glencoe, Ill.: The Free Press, 1958.
27. Hughes, E.C. Professions. In K.S. Lynn & the Eds. of Daedalus (Eds.), *The professions in America.* Boston: Houghton Mifflin, 1965.
28. Hughes, E.C. The social significance of professionalization. In H.W. Vollmer & D.L. Mills (Eds.), *Professionalization.* Englewood Cliffs, N.J.: Prentice-Hall, 1966.
29. Jones, F.E. Social origins in four professions: A comparative study. *International Journal of Comparative Sociology,* 1976, *17*(3-4), 143-163.
30. Kaufman, M. *American medical education: The formative years 1765-1910.* Westport, Conn.: Greenwood Press, 1976.
31. Klegon, D. The sociology of professions: An emerging perspective. *Sociology of Work and Occupations,* 1978, *5*(3), 259-283.
32. Kornhauser, W. The interdependence of professions and organizations. In H.W. Vollmer & D.L. Mills (Eds.), *Professionalization.* Englewood Cliffs, N.J.: Prentice-Hall, 1966.
33. Lopata, H.Z. Expertization of everyone and the revolt of the client. *The Sociological Quarterly,* 1976, *17*(4), 435-447.
34. Moore, W.E. *The professions: Roles and rules.* New York: Russell Sage Foundation, 1970.
35. Parsons, T. Professions. In *International encyclopedia of the social sciences* (Vol. 12). New York: Macmillan Company and The Free Press, 1968.
36. Reader, W.J. *Professional men: The rise of the professional classes in nineteenth-century England.* London: Weidenfeld and Nicolson, 1966.
37. Ritti, R.R., Ference, T.P., & Goldner, F.H. Professions and their plausibility: Priests, work, and belief systems. *Sociology of Work and Occupations,* 1974, *1*(1), 24-51.
38. Roberts, K.L. Nursing: Profession or pretender? *Australian Nurses Journal,* 1980, *9*(10), 33-35; 51.

39. Rosenstein, A.B. The future of education for the professions. *Education Digest*, December 1978, pp. 2-6.

40. Rosenstein, A.B. *The national professions foundation and the future quality of national life.* Paper presented at the annual meeting of the American Association for the Advancement of Science, Houston, Texas, January 5, 1979.

41. Ross, D. Professionalism and the transformation of American social thought. *Journal of Economic History,* 1978, *38,* 494-499.

42. Roth, J. Professionalism: The sociologist's decoy. *Sociology of Work and Occupations,* 1974, *1*(1), 6-23.

43. Schein, E.H. *Professional education: Some new directions.* New York: McGraw-Hill, 1972.

44. Simpson, R.L., & Simpson, I.H. Women and bureaucracy in the semi-professions. In A. Etzioni (Ed.), *The semi-professions and their organization: Teachers, nurses, social workers.* New York: The Free Press, 1969.

45. Strauss, A. *Professions, work, and careers.* New Brunswick, N.J.: Transaction Books, 1975.

46. Strauss, G. Professionalism and occupational associations. *Industrial Relations,* 1963, *2*(3), 7-31.

47. Taylor, L. *Occupational sociology.* New York: Oxford University Press, 1968.

48. Vollmer, H.W., & Mills, D.L. (Eds.). *Professionalization.* Englewood Cliffs, N.J.: Prentice-Hall, 1966.

49. Wilensky, H. The professionalization of everyone. *American Journal of Sociology,* 1964, *70*(2), 137-158.

6

RECAPITULATION AND REDIRECTION WITH EXPLICIT BELIEFS ABOUT NURSING

Where do we go from here? Within all of those references summoned in Section Two, is there a meaningful model for nursing to measure against, aspire to, and take direction from? Or for us as nurses to call upon in negotiating the day-to-day business of survival and growth and caring?

Reading this material must have sparked a feeling of *déjà vu* among those of us who have already completed our basic nursing "schooling." Surely we can recall—some with pride, some with skepticism, and some with tedium—the lists of "criteria for a profession" we were subjected to as students in professional history-trends-or-issues courses. These academic exercises are generally in two parts. First, the hallmarks of professionalism are enumerated; then, nursing is checked against the list. It is like taking a professional inventory.

Commonly cited as requisites for an occupation to claim professional status are:

Extensive university education
A unique body of knowledge

An orientation of service to others
A professional society
Autonomy and self-regulation, sometimes simplistically reduced
to a code of ethics

From an educator's point of view, it would be of interest to determine the long-range effects of these didactic drills on each learner. Even now, the emotion evoked in us by the memory is worth noting. The energy that has been and continues to be consumed in the debates on nursing's professionalism, if converted into electricity, would probably heat, cool, and light our nursing schools for eternity.

To encapsulate our rating, we could take a quick look at one outside and one inside evaluation. Etzioni and other sociologist colleagues have flatly relegated us to the semi-professions (4). Bernhard and Walsh, both nurses, have graphed our progress on the Pavalko professionalism continuum (page 30) like a rather healthy looking flow chart, giving us top scores on social values, motivation, and ethics, and successively lower scores on community, autonomy, education, commitment, and theory (1:10).

As I see it, nursing has scored moderately well in these appraisals, except on the standards relating to a scientific knowledge base and to self-control. Controversy still simmers and erupts over those two issues. In relation to the other criteria, however, nursing seems to have passed muster. We have been in the universities since the early part of the century. There has been a professional society, now called the American Nurses' Association (ANA), since 1897, although it has not yet captured the loyalty of the majority of nurses. In addition, we have long had a code of ethics in successive editions, at one time having appeared on the reverse side of our ANA membership cards for ready reference in times of moral dilemma. As to purpose, nursing's service nature is unimpeachable.

I question, though, whether these professional inventories have done much to aid us in self-development and self-understanding. For with this approach, the emphasis is more on the profession than its members, and, as has been implied, I believe the seeds of professional reformation lie in the individual. Moreover, even when we examine the profession as a whole, strict attention to these checklists seems to bear little fruit or prospect.

Overall, in engaging in these assessments, I have always been left with the rational conclusion that we passed inspection, but with the visceral reaction that something vital has been missed or miscalculated in the inventory.

Frankly, just as I was not inspired by all of this in my student or early practice days, I experienced not a single "Aha, that's for me!" in all the literature surveyed and summarized in the preceding sections. Nevertheless, the search was not in vain. These readings constitute the raw material to which we can apply our creativity and experience as we develop our own model of professionalism for nursing and professionhood for ourselves.

A MODEL FOR NURSING

Could we begin this model-building endeavor with an assumption that whatever nursing is now—and that we won't debate—we need to, and can, do more to improve our condition. It is not necessary to belabor this point with extensive documentation. Public criticism, internal conflict, chronic complaints of powerlessness, attrition from the field, economic injustices—these and other factors all attest that nursing falls somewhere short of perfection. Certainly, this can be said of other occupations as well, but *our* essential concern is nursing. In our numbers and in our services, we are a vast resource for social betterment. Yet our space in the sociopolitical landscape adds up to far less than the sum of our parts. Stated another way, our power is more potential than actual; we are a *potentialized,* rather than an *actualized,* profession.

Also, when our power *is* unleashed, too often it seems to be without clear direction. For example, nursing and the votes it represents have long been well respected by Congress. We have been able to overturn presidential vetoes and rescissions when other seemingly more influential lobbies have failed. But lacking a clear sense of unity or priority on some major issues, such as funding for education or research, we have succeeded in getting a modest amount for everything, instead of an adequate amount for what is most important. Our tentativeness, too, may partially account for the regrettable fact that our presence at the policy tables in all levels of government and in the health industry, with some notable exceptions, is mere tokenism, having recently progressed beyond our earlier stage of invisibility.

This uncertainty is manifest in the clinical setting as well. Having successfully negotiated with employing agencies for professional standards committees, we often cannot seem to identify what measures make the greatest difference in patient care.

These illustrations bring us back to the assumption that, whatever we are in nursing now and notwithstanding the advances we have made, we need to do better. If pursuit of the traditional model of professionalism has not secured for us our proper place in society, what is the model that would move us toward that goal?

Actualization

Consider this alternative: instead of setting our sights on an external ideal—professionalism—and the set of qualifications associated with that ideal, let us compete for the best within ourselves—that is, to be the best we can be in accomplishing the purposes we set out for ourselves. In other words, let us aim to be *self-actualized professionals* forming an *actualized profession*. Granted, these sound like buzzwords; perhaps another brace of terms might be more appealing. By whatever name, however, the pressing need is to stretch our capacities, to stretch our achievements, and to stretch our rewards, both tangible and intangible. In so doing, we will be developing our fullest potentialities in all respects.

We cannot nor should we be satisfied with what we are, rather we must compete for what we can be. James Mac-Gregor Burns, a social philosopher, has identified leadership of two types: transactional and transforming (2). The latter goes beyond meeting existing need and demand to tap potential motives, to satisfy higher needs, and to engage the full person of the follower. Transforming leadership incites "the revolution of rising expectations"—a stirring summons (3:48). In this sense, self-actualization and actualization mean, respectively, engaging the fullness of each of us in the fullness of nursing, the fullness being the most that can be. All of this implies *a deep and abiding awareness of purpose and direction in place of a specific set of objectives or standards*, which is inherently limited by today's vision. Undoubtedly, we can exceed that which we now conceive to be our maximum effort and achievement.

BELIEFS ABOUT NURSING

Within this proffered model, *actualization* and *self-actualization* are seen to stem from clear and consistent direction, and *direction* to stem from *belief*. Thus, first and foremost, WE NEED A BELIEF SYSTEM, an explicit belief system, a manifesto, a social contract. And here I may disappoint you, because I shall not go on to add an existential "to each his own" in this regard. Admittedly, we all operate on an individual set of beliefs, whether known or unknown to us. But nursing, as a professional community, must have and hold a common, recitable ideology just as nations have their constitutional preambles and pledges of allegiance, fraternal societies have their oaths, religions have their creeds. Individualization occurs not in the fundamental tenets that bind the group, but in the translation of them into personal meaning, application, and nuance.

A BELIEF ABOUT BELIEF

Over the decades, nursing, usually with the education establishment in the lead, has seen fit to identify a fundamental *source* from which all thought and action emanated and by which our boundaries are determined. Terminology has changed, and the general conception of that source has undergone repeated modifications. It is difficult to determine to what extent this path has been one of evolution and refinement or faddism. Nevertheless, each generation produces and claims its own mutation, and each evidences a vast discrepancy between the most relaxed and the most restricted construction of the reigning concept.

Within my memory, we have somewhat sequentially committed

ourselves in this regard to *philosophy and purpose, theory* (in an early, impure use of the word), *conceptual framework,* and to a relatively new addition (which is characteristically becoming more amorphous as it gains in popularity)—that of *paradigm.* Listing these variants in this manner is not to suggest falsely an interchangeability among them, but rather to indicate that all have been used at one time or other to contain beliefs and assumptions, though of different levels and classes. Of most significance is that the explication of *source*—the fundamental origin and boundary of nursing thought and activity—is a lasting and important responsibility for the profession.

To meet the most basic level of this need, I commend a direct statement of belief for its simplicity, fundamentality, compatibility, stability, durability, and universality. Let me explain these properties. First, a statement of belief is not inconsistent with other more elaborate and sophisticated efforts to define source and structure as they develop over time. In fact, if one were to consider nursing's foundation as constructed in layers, a simple statement of belief, incorporating conviction about our social contract and essential nature, can be seen as underlying all the rest.

Also, it seems fitting that the form for expressing this source be as basic, fundamental, and enduring as its content. There are few words in our tongue as ageless, common, simple, and true as *belief.* It stands out as exquisitely undefiled within the verbal corruption of any age or place.

Finally, there is the undeniable, though sometimes bothersome, realization that we must communicate, not only among ourselves but with the world around us. When we spout our peculiar brand of *esoterica,* outsiders, depending on mood and circumstance, may be confused, angry, amused, or impressed—but seldom enlightened. One of the most difficult challenges I have faced is speaking for the news media. My language must be laundered several times, with their teasing assistance, before it strikes interviewers as anything but gibberish.

So, who is presumptuous enough to abstract a contemporary set of nuclear beliefs for the profession? Well, I am willing to propose a first draft, declaring twenty-five years in nursing as my only right to do so. During this quarter century, it has been my impression that nursing, to an unfortunate extent, has fallen prey to the tendencies of the emerging professions identified earlier, that is, paying exaggerated attention to the traditional symbols of professionalism and losing sight of original purpose. Whether in the pursuit of academic respectability, or a deeper commitment to securing a firm scientific foundation for practice, or both, we in nursing have devalued the service ideal to raise an intellectual one. We have forgotten that in a profession, as opposed to a basic academic discipline, the latter exists ultimately to serve the former. Thus, in some instances, we have seemed to thrash about, theorizing on quicksand. Most of us now recognize that if we are to regain our footing, *we must reinstate the service ideal in its proper primary relationship to our science and practice, on the one hand, and to our legitimate claims to self-determination and reward, on the other.* This perspective must emerge within the tenets of a balanced ideology, which I have attempted to embody in the following statement.

DECLARATION OF BELIEF
ABOUT THE NATURE AND PURPOSE OF NURSING

I. I believe in nursing as an *occupational force for social good,* a force that, in the *totality of its concern* for all human health states and for mankind's responses to health and environment, provides a distinct, unique, and vital perspective, value orientation, and service.

II. I believe in nursing as a *professional discipline,* requiring a sound education and research base grounded in its own science and in the variety of academic and professional disciplines with which it relates.

III. I believe in nursing as a *clinical practice,* employing particular physiological, psychosocial, physical, and technological means for human amelioration, sustenance, and comfort.

IV. I believe in nursing as a *humanistic field,* in which the fullness, self-respect, self-determination, and humanity of the nurse engage the fullness, self-respect, self-determination, and humanity of the client.

V. I believe that nursing's *maximum contribution* for social betterment is dependent on:
   A. The well-developed *expertise* of the nurse;
   B. The *understanding, appreciation,* and *acknowledgment* of that expertise by the public;
   C. The organizational, legal, economic, and political *arrangements* that enable the full and proper expression of nursing values and expertise;
   D. The ability of the profession to maintain *unity* within diversity.

VI. I believe in *myself* and in my *nursing colleagues:*
   A. In our *responsibility* to develop and dedicate our minds, bodies, and souls to the profession that we esteem and the people whom we serve;
   B. In our *right* to be fulfilled, to be recognized, and to be rewarded as highly valued members of society.

FROM BELIEF TO DIRECTION

Such *beliefs,* short and simple as they may seem, can serve as vectors for nursing by providing both impetus and direction to the profession. We might prove this to ourselves by selecting a small number of nursing issues, dilemmas, or problems and see if, in reading carefully, we cannot find guidance within this ideology.

For example, collective bargaining—its purposes and forms, its merits and demerits—is currently a major controversy in nursing's bubbling crucible. Several of the beliefs impinge on this question, but most specifically those averring that nursing's maximum contribution is dependent on "the organizational, legal, economic, and political arrangements that enable the full and proper expression of nursing values and expertise" and that of "the ability of the profession to maintain unity within diversity." It follows then that collective bargaining is one possible means whereby nursing's competence can be asserted. Yet, if adopted, it must be accomplished in such a way as not to divide the profession; nursing, as a collective, must be organized to assure that cohesiveness is not thus impaired. Also, to refer again to the beliefs, our right "to be rewarded as highly valued members of society" may have to be gained, in some instances, through collective action, such as unionism.

As a second example of beliefs providing direction, let us look at the continuing debate about levels or categories of nursing practice and the respective educational preparation and legal credential for each. (These controversies will be discussed in Chapter 18.) If we subscribe to the second, third, and fourth declarations on the multifaceted nature of nursing and on the conditions essential for our greatest impact to be felt, we must almost necessarily conclude that the practice of an occupation that broadly combines scientific, technological, and humanistic elements might well encompass dual levels of practice. We could further deduce that a significant, though varying, liberal and specific education base would be required for each; that the education/practice/credentialing system that derives should be comprehensible to our various publics; and that organized nursing should bind these elements together.

A third and clinical extrapolation from this ideology could be made to the persistent question of nurses being assigned to areas and responsibilities in hospitals and other work environments for which they have not been prepared by special education or even by on-the-job orientation and experience. Statements II and III, that nursing is too complex in its science and technology to expect all nurses to be proficient in all aspects, render such a practice socially irresponsible, except in the most extenuating and nonrepetitive circumstances. And the assertion that the organizational setting should recognize and capitalize on our expertise makes clear that we must not give sympathy to any claim that employing agencies are powerless to reform in this regard.

This declaration of belief has stood the test of these examples, giving added credence to the promise that an appropriate model for nursing should stem from an ideology or manifesto as proposed, providing general direction for professional policy and action. And development along these lines should also lead toward actualization for the profession and self-actualization of its members. This encourages us to proceed by asking how this direction could be extracted and displayed in a comprehensive, consistent manner. The next chapter suggests a way of accomplishing this.

7

A FRAMEWORK FOR DEDUCING
DIRECTION FROM BELIEF

Having looked at just three applications of the proposed ideology, let's now seek an overall framework within which to extract direction from belief throughout the nursing universe. There are any number of ways to organize our mind's eye view of nursing for this purpose. And since this is an arbitrary decision and not a search for truth, one framework should be as good as another, as long as it works—that is, if it is appropriate, comprehensive, and not unduly complicated. My best attempt, for the moment, and not original, would be to modify the classical education triad of learner-discipline-society into *the individual* nurse, *the practice and the profession* of nursing, and *the social context* of the field as the three spheres of the nursing universe:

NURSING UNIVERSE

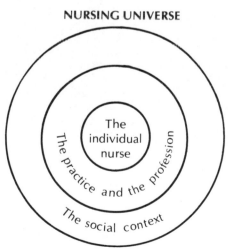

The boundaries between the three concentric spheres have been logically but nevertheless arbitrarily determined and are subject to redefinition after closer scrutiny and application. The *individual* nurse includes students and practitioners, their beliefs and characteristics, and is the core of the nursing universe. The *practice and the profession* include the service and the special knowledge, competencies, and values required to perform it; the settings within which nursing is developed, taught, and provided; and the professional collective, organized to promote and enhance nursing as a social force. The *social context* includes the other health professions, government, health policy, society in general, and all that surrounds and interacts directly and indirectly with us and our practice.

The next step would be to derive directions within each of these three spheres from the previously cited beliefs. For convenience and testing, a grid or matrix can be developed for the insertion of directions emanating from beliefs within the three spheres of the nursing universe. It would look like this:

Text continued on p. 73.

DIRECTION FROM BELIEFS
IN THREE SPHERES OF THE NURSING UNIVERSE

Articles of belief	Spheres of nursing universe		
	Individual*	Practice and the profession†	Social context‡
I. I believe in nursing as an *occupational force for social good,* a force that, in the *totality of its concern* for all human health states and for mankind's responses to health and environment, provides a distinct, unique, and vital perspective, value orientation, and service.	*Includes students and practitioners, their beliefs and characteristics.	†Includes the service and the special knowledge, competencies, and values required to perform it; the settings within which nursing is developed, taught, and provided; and the professional collective, organized to promote and enhance nursing as a social force.	‡Includes the other health professions, government, health policy, society in general, and all that surrounds and interacts directly and indirectly with us and our practice.

Continued.

67

DIRECTION FROM BELIEFS
IN THREE SPHERES OF THE NURSING UNIVERSE—cont'd

Articles of belief	Spheres of nursing universe		
	Individual*	Practice and the profession†	Social context‡
II. I believe in nursing as a professional discipline, requiring a sound education and research base grounded in its own science and in the variety of academic and professional disciplines with which it relates.		*Combined with beliefs III and IV recognizes that nursing is science, humanism, and technology— suggesting dual levels of education and practice.* *The combination further suggests that nurses cannot be used interchangeably because of the breadth and depth of practice.*	

Continued.

III. I believe in nursing as a *clinical practice* employing particular physiological, psychosocial, physical, and technological means for human amelioration, sustenance, and comfort.

DIRECTION FROM BELIEFS
IN THREE SPHERES OF THE NURSING UNIVERSE—cont'd

Articles of belief	Spheres of nursing universe		
	Individual*	Practice and the profession†	Social context‡
IV. I believe in nursing as a *humanistic field*, in which the fullness, self-respect, self-determination, and humanity of the nurse engage the fullness, self-respect, self-determination, and humanity of the client.			

70

V. I believe that nursing's *maximum contribution for social betterment is dependent* on:

A. The well-developed *expertise of the nurse*

B. The understanding, *appreciation, and acknowledgment of that expertise by the public*

C. The organizational, legal, economic, and political *arrangements that enable the full and proper expression of nursing values and expertise*

D. The ability of the *profession to maintain unity within diversity*

Our educational/practice/credentialing system must be comprehensible.

Collective bargaining is justified if it is the best or only arrangement for gaining full expression of nursing's competence.

When collective bargaining is adopted, it must not impair the wholeness or integrity of the profession.

To aid us in fulfilling our social contract, the public must understand how we are educated and what nurses have to offer in values and services.

Continued.

71

DIRECTION FROM BELIEFS
IN THREE SPHERES OF THE NURSING UNIVERSE—cont'd

Articles of belief	Spheres of nursing universe		
	Individual*	Practice and the profession†	Social context‡
VI. I believe in *myself* and in *my nursing colleagues*			
A. In our *responsibility* to develop and dedicate our minds, bodies, and souls to the profession that we esteem and the people whom we serve			
B. In our *right* to be fulfilled, to be recognized, and to be rewarded as highly valued members of society		*Collective bargaining is justified if it is the best or only way to gain these rights without jeopardizing others.*	

72

While I have claimed that the framework is comprehensive, meaning that every issue, every problem, and every dilemma *can* be examined within it and receive direction from it, I shall not tax its capacities in this volume. Nor should anyone. This would involve long and potentially divisive debates on the appropriateness, fit, order, and magnitude of the entries, all of which would be unnecessary because this is intended as a dynamic, working schema. We have our entire professional lives in which to fill it in.

For illustrative purposes the three applications of the ideology from Chapter 6 have been inserted. Let us also note that those general "directions" relating to the *individual* would constitute the attributes for *professionhood*, the concept introduced in Chapter 2 to be discussed in greater detail in Section Five. As we move through the book and deduce further directions from these beliefs, the utility of the framework as a simple device for plotting a course of action for nursing will be seen.

8

THE RELATIONSHIP OF THE IDEOLOGICALLY BASED ACTUALIZATION MODEL TO PROFESSIONALISM

A summary

You may be wondering, "What is the relationship of all of this to the work on professionalism?" Perhaps a summary will help to tie up loose ends, as well as prepare for that which is to come.

First, I advanced the notion that casting nursing's destiny within the classical lists of criteria for a profession has profited us very little, if at all. The professionalism ideal has come under attack in recent years as too self-serving in its motivation and too traditional in its approach. But my chief reason for suggesting that we move beyond it to another model is that I find it inadequate and simplistic for this day and age. It is reactive, rather than active; it forces us to fashion ourselves after an outside, and possibly outmoded, image. Further, it centers on the character of the profession and not of its members.

I went on to propose that we substitute in its place a dynamic, internal ideal—that of actualization, meaning that, with outwardly spiraling aspirations, capacities, and returns

Belief ———→ Direction

to others and ourselves, we would engage the fullness of ourselves in the fullness of nursing.

Then I expressed the conviction that this growth and progress must be anchored in an explicit ideology and that the formulation of belief about our essential nature and purpose is an urgent, collective, and ongoing task for the profession and for its members. This ideology I have variously referred to as a declaration of belief, a manifesto, and a social contract. Whatever the title of the whole, the contents remain *beliefs*.

I then proceeded to illustrate how a proposed set of central beliefs would provide direction for us, suggesting for this analysis that we consider nursing within three concentric spheres of activity: the individual, the practice and the profession, and the social context.

For those who are more visually oriented, the model—pointing out that belief leads to general direction, which in turn leads to the fullest expression of the nurse, and in the aggregate to the fullest expression of nursing—might be depicted something like this:

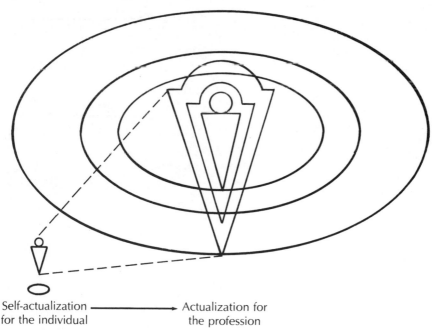

Self-actualization ———————————→ Actualization for
for the individual   the profession

If we wanted to reduce all of this to one short, short summary, it would be:

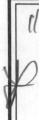

> **Our intent that nursing become its utmost and that we as nurses become our utmost would be better served by a set of internal beliefs about nursing than a set of external criteria about professions.**

REFERENCE LIST FOR SECTION THREE

1. Bernhard, L.A., & Walsh, M. Leadership: The key to the *professionalization of nursing.* New York: McGraw-Hill, 1981.
2. Burns, J.M. *Leadership.* New York: Harper & Row, 1978.
3. Burns, J.M. True leadership. *Psychology Today,* October 1978, pp. 46-58, 110.
4. Etzioni, A. *The semi-professions and their organization.* New York: Free Press, 1969.

THE MEANING OF OUR WORK

9

AN EYE ON THE KALEIDOSCOPE

From the most primitive of beginnings,
man has hunted as relentlessly and
unceasingly for explanations concerning
the meaning of life as he has sought
food and shelter. This never-ending quest
reflects . . . the need to alleviate man's
existential terrors by finding a purpose
for being.

FREDERICK HERZBERG (12:ix)

[Man's] work . . . gives him a secure place
in a portion of reality, in the human
community.

SIGMUND FREUD (8:xx)

To choose a work vocation is to accept
two sets of historical bonds: the bonds
that tie our biographies to ongoing natural
history, and the bonds that link our fate
to man's collective history. Both sets of
bonds disclose human labor as the means
for exploring what we can become—
through our participation in the history
of natural events and through reciprocal
relations among men. To choose a form
of work for our own is, then, to choose our
history; for work defines our biographies,
not as linear behaviors, but as a
convoluted web of shared bonds between
men, and between men and nature.

LOUIS SCHAW (22:xi)

For man, unlike any other thing organic
or inorganic in the universe, grows
beyond his work, walks up the stairs
of his concepts, emerges ahead of
his accomplishments.

JOHN STEINBECK (23:164)

Have you worked well?

[August Rodin's customary greeting] (16:24)

I am not Shakespeare and I am not Hegel,
but I have produced my works with as
much care as I could. Some have been
failures, surely: others less so, and others
have succeeded. That is enough.

JEAN-PAUL SARTRE (21:4)

I was constantly astonished by the
extraordinary dreams of ordinary
people. . . . Those we call ordinary are
aware of a sense of personal worth—or
more often the lack of it—in the work
they do.

STUDS TERKEL (24:xxix-xxx)

Most of us are looking for a calling, not
a job. Most of us . . . have jobs that are too
small for our spirit. Jobs are not big
enough for people.

STUDS TERKEL (24:xxix)

Is it any wonder that in . . . surreal circumstances, status rather than the work itself becomes important. Thus the prevalence of euphemisms in work as well as in war. The janitor is a building engineer; the garbage man, a sanitary engineer. . . . They are not themselves ashamed of their work, but society, they feel, looks upon them as a lesser species. So they call upon promiscuously used language to match the "respectability" of others, whose jobs may have less social worth than their own.

STUDS TERKEL (24:xx)

Picasso can point to a painting. A writer can point to a book. What can I point to? . . . Everybody should have something to point to.

STEELWORKER (24:2)

I don't know who the guy is who said there is nothing sweeter than an unfinished symphony.
. . . But what if he had to create this Sistine Chapel a thousand times a year. Don't you think that would even dull Michelangelo's mind? Or if da Vinci had to draw his anatomical charts thirty, forty, fifty, sixty . . . a hundred times a day? Don't you think that would even bore da Vinci?

STEELWORKER (24:9)

The profession is more likely to be a
terminal occupation. Members do not
care to leave it, and a higher proportion
assert that if they had it to do over
again, they would again choose that type
of work.

GOODE (9:903)

[Nursing] is the most incredibly rich
profession I know of. Would I do it
again? Anytime.

NURSE (13:95)

Nursing is a love-hate thing with me.

NURSE (13:90)

[I] can't live with nursing and can't live
without it.

NURSE (13:90)

I spend half my time defending the
profession and the other half deriding
it.

NURSE (13:95)

Nursing is next to my God and my
husband in my heart.

NURSE (14:116)

84

When I entered nursing . . . I had this
wonderful desire to help people—real
compassion and concern. Even today, I'm
not a cold, uncaring nurse, just a super
busy one with no time to give of myself.

NURSE (14:119)

When I was satisfied with my job,
money seemed less important. Now it's
the only positive reward I get.

NURSE (15:89)

My friend left nursing to become a
waitress. She earns more now in 35
hours than she used to in 40.

NURSE (15:90)

Nursing is not a profession. Check
salaries and status, vis-à-vis the true
professions—law, medicine, education.
We're only considered professional when
it benefits the institution.

NURSE (13:95)

The operative word . . . is *profession.*
Theoretically the professional nurse
defines and employs nursing
intervention; in reality, though, her
judgment counts for very little. The
doctors and administrators make the
real decisions.

NURSE (13:95)

My biggest frustration was that, because
of the attitudes of the doctors at our
hospital, I couldn't practice nursing the
way it should be practiced.

NURSE (15:91-92)

I usually take the authority and do what
I feel is right. My decisions have never
been questioned, but my authority to
make the decision has.

NURSE (14:118)

You love nursing but *not* the conditions under which you have
to practice it. And what you want above all—more than anything
that would benefit you personally—is *the chance to be better
nurses.*

MARJORIE GODFREY (14:95)

Thus, we have heard from others some magnificent
thoughts about the meaning of work. What about ourselves?
In the ideology of an earlier chapter we said:

"I believe in nursing . . . ."
"I believe in myself . . . ."

Nursing and myself. What of the confluence of the two?
How do we satisfy the existential drive to find personal
meaning through our particular human labor?

Examining and deepening our relationship to our profession involves knowing nursing in both a subjective and objective way: Knowing how we experience our vocation. Knowing how it is perceived and defined by others. And achieving a successful integration of these inner and outer worlds.

We could think of this search for meaning as keeping a vigilant eye on the kaleidoscope. As children our hearts quickened as we squinted timorously into that mysterious, shadowy tube, which marvelously burst into bits of colored glass. With the smallest turn of the hand, we created endless, brilliant, variegated patterns. For us, as adults and as professionals, the kaleidoscope represents both the *fragments* within our professional universe—some bright, some dull; some soft, some sharp; some large, some small; some intimate, some remote—and the conceptual *organization,* which combines them into shape and significance. (The difficulty is that we are simultaneously the eye, the hand, the fragment. We see meaning; we give meaning; we are part of meaning. All three we must attend to, else we are the tumbling fragment in a foreign hand.)

Section Three proposed one model capable of adding rationality and perspective to limitless, mutable fragments, thus giving form to nursing. This section brings out for inspection some, just some, of the fragments that float within our vocational kaleidoscope, useless and frustrating, until anchored within a mosaic of relationship and significance. Some of the pieces—those residing within the innermost, the nurse, circle of the nursing universe—are exclusively our own. Others—those within the middle and outer rings of the profession and practice and the social context—are the common property of us all. Yet each fits into the meaning of our work. In this exploration, we'd best begin in the next chapter with our surroundings, with what others have had to say about nursing, and then move inward in the following segment to examine our private worlds and what nursing means to us.

10

NURSING AS
OTHERS FIND IT

A responsible, socially aware profession such as nursing engages continually in self-study and renewal. So, too, do responsible, socially aware members of that profession—in this instance ourselves. Possibly the perceptions of nursing held by those both within and outside the profession will help us to shape our own perceptions and to develop our own sense of what it is to be a nurse.

In this chapter we dip into the deep literary well that reveals how others have defined, characterized, experienced, hoped for, and theorized about nursing. Let us start with the *impersonal* or *objective* aspects relating to definition and conclude with the *personal* or *subjective* aspects relating to job satisfaction and motivation.

DEFINING NURSING: ITS GOALS, CHARACTER, SCOPE

On our bookshelves, next to the catalog of lists of criteria for professionalism, may be several dusty volumes on definitions of nursing. Explicit delineations of its nature and scope exist in law, in the myriad and diverse position statements promulgated by nursing organizations, in bureaucratic policies, and in theories of nursing. A representation from these sources might be introduced here, with recognition of the fact that definitions serve different purposes and accordingly contain different elements.

As defined by law

Superseding all others, in that they are guardians of the public safety and gatekeepers to practice, are the statutory boundaries prescribed in nursing practice acts. The American Nurses' Association, in a recent publication, has suggested this definition for incorporation in state legislation:

> The practice of nursing means the performance for compensation of professional services requiring substantial specialized knowledge of the biological, physical, behavioral, psychological, and sociological sciences and of nursing theory as the basis for assessment, diagnosis, planning, intervention, and evaluation in the promotion and maintenance of health; the casefinding and management of illness, injury, or infirmity; the restoration of optimum function; or the achievement of a dignified death. Nursing practice includes but is not limited to administration, teaching, counseling, supervision, delegation, and evaluation of practice and execution of the medical regimen, including the administration of medications and treatments prescribed by any person authorized by state law to prescribe. Each registered nurse is directly accountable and responsible to the consumer for the quality of nursing care rendered. (2:6)

At the crest of the new wave in legal definition is the 1978 New York State statute, which states:

> "Diagnosing" in the context of nursing practice means that identification of and discrimination between physical and psychosocial signs and symptoms essential to effective execution and management of the nursing regimen. Such diagnostic privilege is distinct from a medical diagnosis.
> "Treating" means selection and performance of those therapeutic measures essential to the effective execution

and management of the nursing regimen, and execution of any prescribed medical regimen.

"Human responses" means those signs, symptoms, and processes which denote the individual's interaction with an actual or potential health problem.

The practice of the profession of nursing as a registered professional nurse is defined as diagnosing and treating human responses to actual or potential health problems, through such services as case finding, health teaching, health counseling, and provision of care supportive to or restorative of life and well-being, and executing medical regimens prescribed by a licensed or otherwise legally authorized physician or dentist. A nursing regimen shall be consistent with and shall not vary any existing medical regimen. (17)

Both the ANA and the New York State statements stress, the first more directly than the second, the autonomy of nursing with respect to purely nursing concerns and functions. This spirit is in contrast to the more conservative and traditional definition, as exemplified by the current Oklahoma act, which dates back to its adoption in 1953.

The practice of professional nursing means the performance for compensation of any acts, in the observation, care and counsel of the ill, injured or infirm, or in the maintenance of health or prevention of illness of others, or in the supervision and teaching of other personnel, or the administration of medications and treatments, as prescribed by a licensed physician or dentist; requiring substantial specialized judgment and skill based on knowledge and application of the principles of biological, physical, and social science. The foregoing shall not be deemed to include acts of diagnosis or prescription of therapeutic or corrective measures. (19)

As defined by the profession

The professional definitions found in association documents reflect more the goals and purposes of nursing than the limits of practice emphasized in law; they are ultimately tools for self-governance. Thus the ANA, in a 1980 social policy statement on nursing, a booklet that all of us should hold dear in our personal libraries, addressed the social context of nursing, the nature and scope of nursing practice, and specialization in nursing. In the Association's words, their definition "maintains . . . historical orientation [illustrated in the beloved Nightingale and Henderson definitions] and at the same time reflects the influence of nursing theory that is a part of nursing's evolution" (1:9). In chronological sequence, to express this historical path, these definitions are:

Nightingale:

[Nursing is to have] charge of the personal health of somebody . . . and what nursing has to do . . . is to put the patient in the best condition for nature to act upon him. (18:preface; 75)

Henderson:

To assist the individual, sick or well, in the performance of those activities contributing to health or its recovery (or to peaceful death) that he would perform unaided if he had the necessary strength, will or knowledge. And to do this in such a way as to help him gain independence as rapidly as possible. (11:42)

And the Association's contemporary version:

Nursing is the diagnosis and treatment of human responses to actual or potential health problems. (1:9)

The ANA document's reference to modern nursing *theory* points us very appropriately to an additional source of enlightenment on the nature of our work.

As defined by theorists

Theorists serve a vital function at the juncture of the *practice* and the *science* of a profession. They join these two critical elements by laying out, in an organized pattern, the phenomena with which the discipline is concerned. These constructs or models become the frameworks within which nursing practice questions are asked and relevant knowledge is supplied. It is in this manner that the nursing universe can be ordered, studied, and directed.

Thus, theorists define nursing for the purpose of creating a conceptual system out of which will ultimately issue scientific description, prediction, and prescription. Toward these ends, theorists tend to define nursing by its goals, its activities, and its view of man as the central phenomenon of nursing's concern. Sister Callista Roy compares and contrasts these elements of the definitions by two other contemporary theorists, Dorothy Johnson and Martha Rogers, with her own and those of Florence Nightingale and Virginia Henderson to whom earlier reference was made (20:7):

COMPARISON OF MODELS OF NURSING

	Nightingale	Henderson	Johnson	Rogers	Roy
View of man	A passive instrument of nature responding to the same laws whether healthy or sick.	A whole, complete, and independent being who has 14 basic activities: breathe, eat and drink, eliminate, move and maintain posture, sleep and rest, dress and undress, maintain body temperature, keep clean, avoid danger, communicate, worship, work, play, and learn.	A behavioral system composed of 8 subsystems: affiliative, achievement, dependency, aggressive, eliminative, ingestive, restorative, sexual.	A unified whole possessing integrity and manifesting: wholeness, openness, unidirectionality, pattern and organization, sentence and thought.	A biopsychosocial being in constant interaction with a changing environment and having four modes of adaptation: physiologic needs, self-concept, role function, and interdependence.

Continued.

Sister Callista Roy, *Introduction to Nursing: An Adaptation Model,* © 1976, p. 7. Reprinted by permission of Prentice-Hall, Inc., Englewood Cliffs, New Jersey.

COMPARISON OF MODELS OF NURSING—cont'd

	Nightingale	Henderson	Johnson	Rogers	Roy
Goal of nursing	To put man in the best condition for nature to act upon him.	To substitute for what the patient lacks in physical strength, will, or knowledge to make him complete, whole, or independent.	To bring about the patient's behavioral stability.	To promote harmony between man and his environment with the ultimate goal of reaching the highest state of health possible.	To promote adaptation in the four adaptive modes
Nursing activities	"A careful nurse will keep constant watch over her sick." To provide the proper use of fresh air, light, warmth, cleanliness, quiet, and diet.	To know the patient (assessment), identify what patient lacks (diagnosis), help supply this lack (intervention), and evaluate success (evaluation).	To assess behavioral stability, decide on the dynamics of behavioral instability, intervene by restricting, defending, inhibiting, or facilitating, and evaluate resulting patient behavior.	To gather data about man in his environmental field, and to use technical activities, manual skills or human relations to repattern man and the environment.	To assess patient behaviors and factors which influence adaptation level and to intervene by manipulating the influencing factors (focal, contextual, and residual stimuli).

As defined by debate

When viewed in the aggregate, definitions of nursing reflect the uncertainties about its nature. Therefore, another
way to look at the meaning of our work is through these persistent controversies. Nursing is not alone in being subjected
to debate. Surely any profession, in its effort to characterize
and distinguish itself, must give as much attention to that
which is in dispute, as to that which is agreed on. Such coun-
tervailing opinions are the irritants at the growing edge of the
field. In nursing, much of our disaccord is around the very
essential aspects of our practice—tasks and processes, roles
and functions, settings.

We know these disagreements well, for we bump into
them at every turn. Nurse educators and their service counterparts are acutely aware of them, since these discrepant
views are the major source of tensions between the two
groups. It is frequently said the former educate students for a
practice world that does not exist. The academicians counter
that this is true but that they are preparing our professional
progeny to create a better world. This dilemma, in itself, is an
unresolved conflict to be added to those that follow. If we are
not together, then who is to lead? And to whom should we
listen?

It is most striking to list these controversies as extremes,
as I have done with the following. Yet it must be understood
that, overall, both practice and opinion range along these
continua, rather than congregate at the poles. Also, it should
be acknowledged that these attributes do not arrange themselves into neat pairs of opposites but again are arbitrarily
determined.

In traveling down this tentative summary, we might ask

ourselves first, "Is nursing currently more toward one end or the other of the spectrum with respect to the following characteristics and in which direction is it moving?" And then, "Where should nursing be?"—keeping in mind our professional ideology.

Intellectual vs Routine, task-oriented
Dependent vs Independent
Science vs Art, intuition
Psychosocial ("soft" sciences) vs Physical, physiological, technological ("hard" sciences)
Individual care (bedside) vs Coordination, management (deskside)
Creative, innovative vs Repetitive, standardized
Hospital vs Community
Illness care vs Wellness promotion

Do you find these characteristics to be in dispute? How large a problem do these unresolved issues represent? Are there other issues to be added to these?

In drafting our responses and in reviewing all definitions, we may wish to recall two earlier frames of reference that are pertinent here.

First, we could retrieve from the U.S. National Labor Relations Act a description of *professional work,* which, incidentally, is an example of definition by bureaucratic policy:

i. predominantly intellectual and varied in character as opposed to routine mental, manual, mechanical, or physical work;

ii. involving the consistent exercise of discretion and judgment in its performance;

iii. of such a character that the output produced or the result accomplished cannot be standardized in relation to a given period of time;

iv. requiring knowledge of an advanced type in a field of science or learning customarily acquired by a prolonged course of specialized intellectual instruction and study in an institution of higher learning or a hospital, as distinguished from a general academic education or from an apprenticeship or from training in the performance of routine mental, manual, or physical processes. (5:289)

Second, the ideology explicated on page 61 answers several questions in the debate. In effect, it declares that nursing is all of these. For example, the conviction was expressed that nursing is concerned with man in all health states—wherever he may be and in wellness or illness. Nursing was described as scientific, humanistic, and clinical in nature, thus developing and applying its own science, as well as using that of related disciplines, and "employing particular physiological, psychosocial, physical, and technological means for human amelioration, sustenance, and comfort." Ergo, our practice is intellectual and technical, attending to psyche, soma, and social context. Further, the position was taken that conditions in the practice setting must be such as to assure the maximum benefit from nursing's values and expertise. Within this context, professional autonomy is justified on the basis of enabling our greatest contribution to the public welfare, not as a symbol of nor reward for catching the coveted, if tarnished, brass ring of professionalism. Since our freedom is such a heartfelt issue with us, we must save time in a later chapter for a deeper discussion of its meaning.

SATISFACTIONS AND DISSATISFACTIONS

In addition to the impersonal dimensions of definitions discussed in the preceding, nursing also takes its meaning as it is experienced by its practitioners. These are the personal meanings that collect and interact in various ways with less subjective meanings to mold the profession. In moving into this dimension, it becomes apparent that nursing cannot be viewed in any realistic sense as a sterile phenomenon, un-contaminated by the conditions of its practice. When we perceive ourselves at the center of those concentric circles of the nursing universe,

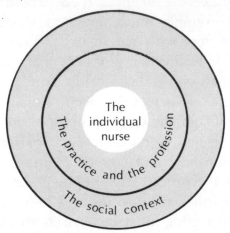

our sense of being hemmed in by larger forces is palpable. On the job, it is even more so. While we recognize our rightful part in shaping those forces, we are, nevertheless, subjected to them.

Although a later chapter discusses specific factors in the work environment, we might consider here, more broadly, the good and the bad of nursing, as reported by those who are engaged in it. The literature yields generously on this subject and we can only lightly tap these references. In doing so, we could consider whether we are in accord or disaccord with those who shared their innermost thoughts with the researchers.

Herzberg's motivation-hygiene theory of job satisfaction has been a popular one for studies of this nature. To become oriented to his approach, we might begin as he did with his original subjects, who were engineers and accountants. We might imagine ourselves before the interviewer, who asks of us:

> Recall a time when you felt particularly good about your job (or, if you are a student, your clinical experiences and observations). Select a circumscribed period in which an identifiable series of events was occurring, not just when you were generally on a psychological high. Describe the events. What made you feel as you did? Did these feelings of satisfaction affect your performance? Your personal relationships? Your well-being?
>
> What was the nature of the sequence of events that served to neutralize or return your attitudes to "normal"?
>
> Think now of a time when you felt negative about your job. Describe the events in that scene. And so forth.

Translating such events as reported by his respondents into factors, Herzberg extracted five that were:

"strong determinants of job satisfaction:
achievement,
recognition,
work itself,
responsibility, and
advancement;

the last three being of
greater importance for
lasting change of attitudes"
(12:72-73).

Herzberg's additional findings were that:

"The major dissatisfiers were:
company policy and administration,
supervision,
salary,
interpersonal relations, and
working conditions" (12:74).

We might ponder these clusters for a few minutes. Are they familiar? Would our experiences fit these patterns? As we compare the lists with each other, do we find anything striking?

Herzberg's most startling discovery was that the satisfiers and dissatisfiers do not stack up as obverse pairs; that is, reversing a satisfier does not create a dissatisfier, or vice versa. Rather, two separate themes. The satisfier grouping relates to what the worker does; the dissatisfier grouping, to the context in which he does it. Because of their nature, the satisfiers have been labeled as *motivators* and the dissatisfiers as *hygiene* or *maintenance* factors. The motivators lead to growth and self-actualization; the maintenance factors lead to unpleasantness, which the individual seeks to avoid.

The dual factor theory has been applied to several nurse populations. One study, conducted by Anderson and reported by Herzberg in verification of his theory, involved staff nurses in a VA Hospital in Utah. *Recognition* and *achievement* turned up as motivators, and *company policy and administration, interpersonal relationships with superiors,* and *working conditions,* as dissatisfiers (12:115).

In 1977, Cronin-Stubbs reviewed five studies based on this theory, including staff nurse and supervisor samples, and added to these the findings from her own research with newly graduated nurses in two Chicago hospitals (7). As is frequently the case when research results are studied, more questions than answers surfaced. But they are interesting questions, prompting further thought about nursing's unique characteristics. For example, Cronin-Stubbs found, contrary to Herzberg's conclusions, that *achievement* was both an important satisfier and dissatisfier for neophyte nurses. When patients improved, nurses felt good; when tasks were not completed successfully, nurses felt bad. *Recognition* from patients, peers, and physicians also led to good feelings to a significant degree. Dissatisfaction resulted from *too much responsibility,* the *incompetence of allied personnel* (a factor not identified by Herzberg's subjects), *poor interpersonal relationships with subordinates* (compared with superiors, as indicated earlier), and *unsatisfactory working conditions.* Surprising? Not really.

Ullrich reported in 1978 that the Herzberg two-factor theory was not upheld when he studied nurses in one hospital in Tennessee. He found dissatisfaction with intrinsic factors, such as achievement and responsibility and the work itself, to be as culpable in causing turnover as the extrinsic factors of technical supervision, hospital policy, and so forth. Additional negative factors, such as interpersonal relations with patients and kin and patients' incurable illnesses, surfaced also. His overall conclusion was that creating an organizational form that matched task requirements with individual aspirations was most important in promoting job enrichment in nursing (25).

From these limited comparisons of nurses with members of other occupational groups and of nurses with nurses, three cautious, interrelated observations about our job attitudes could be made: (1) *the work itself* does not seem to have assumed the positive effects for us that it has for others; (2) work environment appears to loom large in our feelings about our work, perhaps overshadowing work content; and (3) we are a diverse, heterogeneous group with respect to motivation, if the inconsistent findings are to be believed. And, a nagging, incriminating question: Why does *advancement* seldom show up on the nursing lists, either as a satisfier or dissatisfier? Is advancement so foreign to our goals and experience?

Let us make a slight turn in focus, from satisfactions to reward, and an international leap, from this country to the United Kingdom, to learn what we can from Austin's 1977 doctoral dissertation, which investigated *Professionalism and the Nature of Nursing Reward* in Wales (3). There we find support for the contention that nursing is, indeed, fragmented as to the pursuit of reward and, further, that we are, indeed, unlike most professions. As the author summed it up:

> It was found that nurses, for the most part, desired intrinsic rewards for their work and that the high appeal of intrinsic rewards had not been translated into a high desirability for extrinsic rewards—a dynamic common to many professional groups. Finally, this examination of expected work rewards reveals the segmentary nature of nursing. Not only do factors of biography, mobility, work context and dominant work orientation profoundly influence the expectation of given rewards, only very minimally are the extrinsic rewards currently promulgated as legitimate for the profession as a whole by nursing's professional leaders, reflected in the work reward expectations of this sample of nurses. (3:9)

Hence, what leaders want for nursing is not necessarily what practicing nurses want for themselves. The extrinsic rewards promoted by the former are the "given quantities of money, prestige, and power which are affixed to roles and belong to those who occupy the role" (3:14). The 320 staff nurses studied by Austin continued to incline toward the traditional rewards of an intrinsic nature, such as self-esteem, "which persons derive from their work, and vary, to some extent, from individual to individual" (3:14).

There is another interesting way of looking at what nursing means to the individual who practices it, which, in addition to bringing together the earlier content on professionalism and the later discourse on ideology, introduces the subject of motivation. Twenty-five years ago, in conducting a study of general duty nurses for the Missouri Nurses' Association, Habenstein and Christ constructed three nurse-types, summarized in the following profiles.

Professionalizer

The professionalizer nurse had no overriding ideal directing her actions. Her emphasis is not so much on the patient as it is on a base of scientific knowledge and its application. Although not strictly a scientist herself, she feels she must use intellectually-based tools in a professional way to heal. She sees her function to stage manage therapeutic drama.

She expects society to trust her to perform competently but she expects to be judged on this performance only by her fellow professionals. She also believes that her professional status entitles her to certain prerogatives.

Traditionalizer

The traditionalizer nurse has an all encompassing ideal of dedication in the Florence Nightingale tradition. This type of nurse has as her base nursing's role as exemplified in past generations of experience rather than the scientific knowledge base of the professionalizer.

She expects to be judged, not by her colleagues, but by how well her actions match the traditional nursing model of self sacrifice and abnegation of her own personality to the demands of the job.

Utilizer

The utilizer nurse has no predominate motivation or direction-giving ideal to her work. To her, nursing is only "a job". She has little or no personal investment in her work and therefore will not become involved in efforts to improve the status of the profession.

She expects to be judged on how well she does her job as it is specified within the narrowly defined limits of individual tasks. She does not relate her performance of these individual elements to a greater whole. She is uninvolved personally in nursing. (10)

Granted, these are more like caricatures, overdrawn and oversimplified, than true-to-life portraits. And we may wish to quarrel with some features, or to reorganize, or to subdivide them. Nevertheless, they provide food for thought and may have some usefulness in our self-appraisal. If we were to attempt to draw our own sketches for self-understanding using the preceding choices reduced to simplest terms, we might ask ourselves:

> If nursing is (a) tradition, (b) tasks, and (c) knowledge and intellectual activity, the greatest of these is _____.
>
> Professional validation derives from (a) peer approval, (b) the quality of my performance, (c) my superiors in the work place, or (d) completing the tasks of the day's work.
>
> Nursing is (a) a calling, (b) a vehicle for self-development, or (c) a job.
>
> As a nurse, I (a) create and manage a health-promoting, therapeutic environment; (b) uphold traditional standards; or (c) carry out daily prescribed activities.

Measuring ourselves within the dimensions outlined by other observers of the nursing role and character leads us now to closer introspection, to the "I-Nursing Relationship," the most personal meaning of our work.

11

THE I-NURSING RELATIONSHIP

We need to move in. Deeper into the center of the nursing universe. Deeper into ourselves and the meaning we give to and take from our work.

Philosopher Martin Buber, in writing on the world of relation, leads us compellingly into this innermost circle, with his "I consider a tree" passage:

> I can look on it as a picture: stiff column in a shock of light, or splash of green shot with the delicate blue and silver of the background.
>
> I can perceive it as movement: flowing veins on clinging, pressing pith, such of the roots, breathing of the leaves, ceaseless commerce with earth and air—and the obscure growth itself.
>
> I can classify it in a species and study it as a type in its structure and mode of life.
>
> I can subdue its actual presence and form so sternly that I recognise it only as an expression of law—of the laws in accordance with which a constant opposition of forces is continually adjusted, or of those in accordance with which the component substances mingle and separate.
>
> I can dissipate it and perpetuate it in number, in pure numerical relation.
>
> *In all this the tree remains my object, occupies space and time, and has its nature and constitution.*
>
> *It can, however, also come about, if I have both will and grace, that in considering the tree I become bound up in*

relation to it. The tree is now no longer *It.* I have been seized by the power of exclusiveness [emphasis added]. (4:7)

By Buber's definition, primary words do not signify things but suggest relations. They are spoken from the whole being. "The primary word *I-Thou* establishes the world of relation" (4:6).

Four times I have set forth on and aborted this exploration into *the meaning of our work to ourselves.* So many false starts into the most sensitive of all segments are not surprising. Such a search for the personal meaning of vocation demands no less of us than probing around in our self-concepts. Perhaps a textbook approach is best for easing into this delicate subject.

Where and how does nursing fit into our perceptions of our essential being? From the phenomenological point of view, we might visualize our perceptual field as made up of an inner and outer circle. The inner circle, representing the self-concept, contains those generalizations we hold about ourselves; the outer circle represents the environment and our generalizations about it.*

PERCEPTUAL FIELD

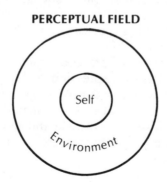

---

*This phenomenological conceptualization draws heavily on the work of Combs and Snygg (6).

The self-concept incorporates and organizes perceptions about myriad aspects of "the real me"; for example, physical appearance, health, intelligence, religion, sexuality, socioeconomic status, personal relationships, values, and on and on. Somewhere within this inner world of perceptions is a sense of purpose. That sense of purpose may, more specifically, be vocation, and vocation may, more specifically, be nursing. Looking penetratingly into our defined self, how do we find nursing? Great or small? Central or peripheral? And what is the motivation behind the place assigned to nursing in this personal world?

These questions may seem strange, but let us pursue this line of thinking. For analytical purposes, we could entertain the idea that *involvement, commitment,* and *motivation* are three separate aspects of the sense of vocation within the self-concept. *Involvement* could be seen as the quantitative measure of life resources, such as time and energy, devoted to the occupation of nursing. *Commitment* could be seen as the intimacy of the perceptions about nursing to the very core of the self. In the proximal or most central relationship, the sense of self and sense of vocation are inseparable, inextricably bound together. Therefore, in the case of extreme commitment, the vocation is the major organizing structure of self. In the distal or peripheral relationship, the profession can be easily detached from the self; it is not essential to the definition of self, as Schaw and Freud saw the case to be (page 81). This imagery comes easily to the nurse quoted in the introduction, "Nursing is next to my God and my husband in my heart" (page 84).

To visualize this distinction between involvement and commitment, we might extract the "self" core from the perceptual field diagrammed previously and note within it the *position* and the *intensity* of the shading that represents the sense of vocation within the self-concept:

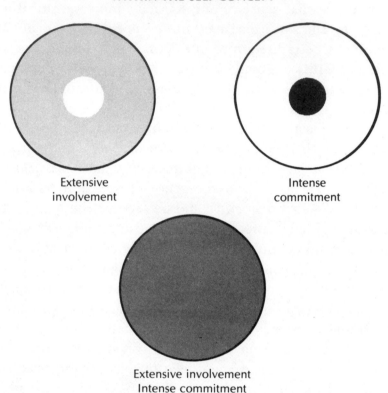

**VOCATIONAL INVOLVEMENT AND COMMITMENT
WITHIN THE SELF-CONCEPT**

Extensive
involvement

Intense
commitment

Extensive involvement
Intense commitment

Motivation, as the third aspect of this sense of vocation, is the driving force—the "what's in it for us?" behind our involvement and commitment.

To grasp possible relationships among these aspects, consider these four sets of circumstances:

Nurse A, solely out of economic necessity, is working full time. Nursing, in consuming a great portion of her time and energy, has forced itself in a big way into her self-concept. Yet she thinks of herself principally as a mother of four children. Nursing is her livelihood, sometimes pleasant, sometimes unpleasant, but overall a distraction from her main vocation. She has no career plans.

The I-Nursing Relationship: Her involvement is great; her commitment is minimal or peripheral; as to motivation, nursing supports her primary interest—her family.

Nurse B had a distinguished career in nursing as an academician until recent years when she has had to greatly reduce her professional responsibilities as a result of impaired health. The activities of daily living require a major portion of her inner resources. First and foremost, she identifies herself as a nurse. Nursing has enabled her to develop her talents and to earn a prominent place in society. Also, it has provided an exciting challenge to her leadership and intellectual capabilities.

The I-Nursing Relationship: Involvement is minimal; commitment is significant or central; motivations are intellectual stimulation and self-enhancement.

Nurse C has found little satisfaction in nursing. She is employed part-time through a registry while she attends a data processing school. She intends to change her career.

The I-Nursing Relationship: Involvement is moderate; commitment is nil, at the very rim of the self-concept, soon to disappear over the edge; as to motivation, nursing is a living until she finds something better.

Nurse D is a full-time student. He has long been interested in a career of a social welfare nature. He selected nursing because he saw it as a tangible expression of his ideal of caring for others. He is somewhat disillusioned because the profession seems to be in a state of turmoil, and he feels caught up in a clash of values—his own, and those of the school, and the clinical environment.

109

The I-Nursing Relationship: Involvement is great; commitment is in flux; motivation is pursuit of the service ideal.

Of course, as we use the schema in an attempt to examine ourselves and others, we quickly realize that nothing so variegated and fluid as a sense of vocation can be analyzed so simply. But this approach serves as a crude instrument for introspection.

For example, as to our *involvement*, we might ask ourselves about the amount of precious life resources of time and energy we devote or intend to devote to nursing. And, irrespective of our time and energy consumed by nursing, what is our *commitment?* To what extent is our self-concept, our very identity, tied up in this vocation? When we are asked to identify ourselves to new acquaintances, do we volunteer proudly or reluctantly, or not at all, that we are nurses?

If nursing is a major part of our lives, what is the *motivating force?* Is nursing for us a livelihood; a vehicle for gaining recognition; a medium for self-expression and achieving excellence; an opportunity to provide a service to others; a distraction from or balance against other aspects of life; an attachment to the wider world outside of family; something else; or a combination of these? On the contrary, if nursing is *not* a major influence in our lives, is it because of the nature of the work, the nature of the circumstances surrounding the work, or the setting in which it occurs? Or the other more important, interesting, or pressing things that dominate our lives? Or is there another explanation?

What brought us into nursing? The dedication as depicted in novels and biographies about nurses? The drama as portrayed on television? Fascination with the presumed content of nursing practice? Family traditions or expectations? A role model? A well-thought-out career plan?

What were we looking for? And what did we find? If there are major discrepancies between the two, how have they influenced our I-Nursing relationship?

What, in fact, is our I-Nursing relationship? This we must forever seek to know and to stengthen.

12

CLOSING THE CIRCLE

"Know thyself" has always been good and sound advice. And that is the message this part of the book is intended to convey. To become self-actualized—that is, to achieve one's fullness, one's professionhood, within a vocation—it is essential to know one's self, one's work, and the bonds that join the two and fuse them with the human community. (Again, the individual, the practice and profession, the social context.)

This process of knowing raises such questions as: What is the content and the scope of nursing? What induced us to seek a career in nursing? What is its significance in our lives? What motivation underlies our commitment to nursing? How do we view the nature of nursing? What do we like about it? What don't we like about it? In these respects, how do we fit into the larger circle of all who share these vocational bonds and constitute our professional collective? This section has touched ever so lightly on these questions in the hope of arousing deeper and more significant self-examination.

And, having delved for these personal understandings within these pages, we might consider now where we stand with those who testified at the outset of Chapter 9.

> These bonds disclose human labor as the means for exploring what we can become. . . . To choose a form of work for our own is, then, to choose our history.

I have produced my work with as much care as I could. That is enough.

Most of us have jobs that are too small for our spirit.

What can I point to?

Nursing is the most incredibly rich profession I know of.

Nursing is a love-hate thing with me.

I love nursing but *not* the conditions under which I practice it.

Would I do it again?

And, having searched with you, I make my own admission that:

Nursing is, for me, an exquisite, excruciating obsession.

And this admission reminds me that those of us who are in the grips of the vision of nursing as a social force dominating and reforming the health scene are like anxious, self-important diamond cutters, circling a giant uncut stone. We argue as to where the cleavage must be made to release its greatest brilliance; hesitant to act lest, through misstroke, the gem be shattered into dull bits of glass, swept into history's dustbin of unfilled promise.

The fallacy in this drama is that there is no giant stone— only myriad smaller ones. It is in each of these—in each of us—that the radiance must be developed throughout each facet.

REFERENCE LIST FOR SECTION FOUR

1. American Nurses' Association. *Nursing: A social policy statement.* Kansas City, Missouri: Author, 1980.
2. American Nurses' Association. *The nursing practice act: Suggested state legislation.* Kansas City, Missouri: Author, 1980.
3. Austin, R. Professionalism and the nature of nursing reward. *Journal of Advanced Nursing,* 1978, 3, 9-23.
4. Buber, M. *I and thou* (2nd ed.). New York: Charles Scribner's Sons, 1958.
5. Cleland, V. The professional model. *American Journal of Nursing,* 1975, 75, 288-292.
6. Combs, A.W., & Snygg, D. *Individual behavior: A perceptual approach to behavior.* New York: Harper & Row, 1959.
7. Cronin-Stubbs, D. Job satisfaction and dissatisfaction among new graduate staff nurses. *Journal of Nursing Administration,* 1977, 7(10), 44-49.
8. Freud, S. Cited in S. Terkel, *Working.* New York: Avon Books, 1975.
9. Goode, W.J. The profession: Reports and opinion. *American Sociological Review,* 1960, 25, 902-904.
10. Habenstein, R.W., & Christ, E.A. *Professionalizer, traditionalizer, and utilizer.* Columbia, Missouri: University of Missouri, 1955.
11. Henderson, V. *Basic principles of nursing care.* London: International Council of Nurses, 1961.
12. Herzberg, F. *Work and the nature of man.* New York: Thomas Y. Crowell Company, 1966.
13. How nurses feel about nursing (Part one). *Nursing 78,* 1978, 8(4), 89-102.
14. How nurses feel about nursing (Part two). *Nursing 78,* 1978, 8(5), 105-119.
15. How nurses feel about nursing (Part three). *Nursing 78,* 1978, 8(6), 81-95.
16. *Lladro: The art of porcelain.* Mallorea and Barcelona: Salvat Editores, S.A., 1979.
17. New York Education Law (McKinney), Article 139, Section 6902 (no date).
18. Nightingale, F. *Notes on nursing.* London: Brandon Systems Press, 1970. (facsimile edition)
19. Oklahoma Nursing Practice Act, 59 O. S. 567.3(b), 1953.
20. Roy, S.C. *Introduction to nursing: An adaptation model.* Englewood Cliffs, N.J.: Prentice-Hall, 1976.
21. Sartre, J.-P. Author-philosopher Sartre dies. In *San Francisco Chronicle,* April 16, 1980, p. 4.

---

22. Schaw, L. *The bonds of work.* San Francisco: Jossey-Bass, 1968.
23. Steinbeck, J. *The grapes of wrath.* New York: Penguin Books, 1939.
24. Terkel, S. *Working.* New York: Avon Books, 1975.
25. Ullrich, R.A. Herzberg revisited: Factors in job dissatisfaction. *Journal of Nursing Administration,* 1978, 8(10), 19-24.

ESSAYS ON THE QUALITIES OF PROFESSIONHOOD

13

DRAWING UP
THE SPECIFICATIONS

The previous section was intended to stimulate the formation of a *gestalt* on "The Meaning of Our Work" by mingling external perspective on the nature of nursing with examination of our own feelings about our vocation. As such, it was entirely descriptive in content and largely oriented in the here and now. This background, which points out the confusion and uncertainty within a profession striving earnestly to progress, may contribute to our readiness now to return to the futuristic, idealistic mode introduced earlier in Chapter 6. We should be prepared to reach out through our beliefs for those individual qualities associated with passage toward professional self-actualization or professionhood for ourselves and consequently toward actualization for nursing.

Although the term "essay" often promises a touch of elegance, there are no such pretensions in this instance. Used here, the word acts simultaneously as a reminder and a disclaimer. This particular literary form—by definition, an interpretative composition dealing with subjects from a limited or personal point of view—constrains me from excessive appeal to other writers and notifies you that the treatment will, indeed, be "limited" and "personal." Limited, in that no effort to catalog and detail all of the virtues advocated for professional persons will be made. Personal, in that I shall speak of those characteristics whereof I am moved to speak, as they seem especially valuable, or lacking, or misunderstood.

Since nursing is such a studied and introspective field— and one suffering overpowering frustrations for which we constantly search for explanations and simple remedies—our literary bank is overflowing with references to both commendable and condemnable traits. These discourses range in tenor from dispassion to diatribe. In fact, we have been so active in generating such prescriptions that it is possible to get bogged down at the foot of the alphabet: accountability, activism, advocacy, aggressiveness, assertiveness, authority, autonomy, and so forth. So, you may ask, who needs another list?

Not another list, but a fresh list or a fresh look at old lists. In either event, a list based on our professional ideology if we are dedicated to acting consistently from such a philosophical base. By collapsing and reordering the core beliefs on page 61 as they related to the individual sphere of the nursing universe, we can formulate this fundamental question: *What attributes are essential in the worker who seeks to serve his fellow man and be self-fulfilled through his eminence in the unique scientific, clinical, humanistic, and collegial health-related field of nursing?* Our specifications should be grounded in this plain bill of particulars in which the moral, ethical, intellectual, and practical dimensions have been accounted for. To specify *less* is to risk failing the mission of the profession; to specify *more* is to chisel a needless stereotype and thus do a disservice to the person, the profession, and the public.

In setting out to identify these cardinal virtues, I have given a lot of thought to earlier efforts of this nature and am impressed with the tendency to mix characteristics of a different order and level. For example, combining traits with habits, beliefs with behaviors, primary qualities with their subsidiaries, means with ends or side effects, and the extrinsic with the intrinsic. I am not at all convinced this shortcoming can be totally avoided, but I do admit to having kept these classification problems in mind in drawing up this modest proposal. Ultimately, I have accepted what has fallen into place in my kaleidoscope (Chapter 9) after considerable reading and contemplation. Those that did not make the list have not been relegated to the undesirable, or even to the unimportant, but appear to fit in a different context.

Reduced to their basics, the qualities I would propose as the bare necessities for professionhood could best be categorized as *attitudes*—attitudes defined as "organismic states of readiness to respond in a characteristic way to a stimulus, as an object, concept, or situation."

The question again: *What attributes are essential in the worker who seeks to serve his fellow man and be self-fulfilled through his eminence in the unique scientific, clinical, humanistic, and collegial health-related field of nursing?*

It seems to me we must hold and manifest these three fundamental attitudes:

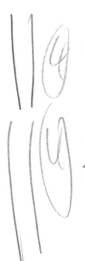

> Social significance—certainty about the nature and importance of our work; sense of mission and social sanction
>
> Ultimacy of performance—commitment to doing our most and our best in our work
>
> Collegiality and collectivity—conviction that responsibility and authority are shared and that the wholeness of the profession must be preserved

These are stated here in what seems to be a logical sequence, not necessarily the order in which they develop in the individual. Ultimacy, since it concentrates on the nursing "task" itself, may be the first to take root in the student of nursing. And, if nurtured, later collegiality and, later still, social significance may bud and blossom. Or, they may not appear at all in any substantial, functional form. This developmental progression of the socialization process would be an interesting subject for future study, but at this point we cannot go beyond this frank conjecture.

14

SOCIAL SIGNIFICANCE

"I believe in nursing as an occupational force for social good" and "I believe in myself" as a valuable member of this occupational force. These two statements are the alpha and the omega of our belief, which, together, form the basis for the sense of *social significance* critical to our professionhood. Social significance, in my view, is the absolute, unwavering, yet realistic conviction about the actual and potential importance of one's work to society. It is the certainty that the world is a better place for having nursing and for having us.

I am speaking here of something deeper, stronger, and more well-defined than the brittle idealism of youth, which may be the precursor to the later, truer, tempered form. It seems to me that this genuine, mature attitude of social significance is created from at least four elements—two *relating to our persons* and two *relating to our profession*—within each of us.

Those *relating to our persons* are embodied in a self-concept that incorporates (1) the *desire* to make a social contribution and (2) the *confidence* that we have the personal capacities to do so. Stated in different terms, we must have a personal *sense of purpose*, sometimes described as role identification, and a *sense of capability* compatible with this service ideal. Those elements *relating to our profession* are similarly embodied in a concept of nursing that incorporates and "professes" (3) the value of its social contribution in a *global* way, as seated in our broad ideology, along with (4) at least a partial picture of its *specific* accomplishments, past, present, and future.

Social significance gives us pride in our calling and in ourselves. Yet it is so easy to lose sight of both significance and pride in the day-to-day rounds of patient care or within the diverse and seemingly disconnected demands of schools of nursing.

If social significance is a critical attribute, we must be concerned about those factors that enter into its development. Three are most easily identified. Certainly, the *educational process* and the learning environment are highly influential in the shaping of the views of the self and of the profession. The presence of a *research* base for nursing, strong enough to offer predictability and credibility to our practice, will give us, and others, added confidence in our social impact. Additionally, as individuals and as a corporate body, we see ourselves reflected in *the eyes of others*, in and outside of nursing. Our colleagues do indeed tell us in numerous, both blatant and subtle, ways what they believe about us, about themselves, and about nursing. And our public image is a major consideration in our sense of social significance. As was acknowledged in our ideology: "I believe that nursing's maximum contribution for social betterment is dependent on . . . the understanding, appreciation, and acknowledgment of [our] expertise by the public." Thus is our community sanction derived and perceived. We are both inwardly and outwardly validated. How we appear in the eyes of others and the image we project are mutually reinforcing. A strong self-concept and a positive personal presence—as seen in the way we dress, the way we carry ourselves, the way we enter a room, the way we present our ideas—can set this cycle into motion.

The key to the preceding, and perhaps at the very heart of social significance, may be the visible consequences of one's work. Chapter 9 recorded the anguished cry of the steelworker, which burst out as he compared his product with that of the artist, "What can I point to? Everyone should have something to point to" (page 83). This bears much, much thought for us in nursing.

You hold in your hand the outcome of my solitary endeavor—a book. Abstract thought has taken on a concrete form. It can be touched, read, and even smelled and tasted, if you were so disposed. It can be studied, stored, retrieved. It can be pointed to. Although its effect on you and others will be difficult to determine, still it can be pointed to.

Before secluding myself in my study to begin this work, I asked a number of graduate students and hospital nurses to jot down on a scrap of paper five words or phrases that came to mind when they thought about the nature of clinical nursing. Responses were scattered—some surprising, some not. The dominant theme was that of *caring*. Caring, of course, is both feeling and its expression. But it is not product or consequence, and the consequence of our ministrations is often obscure or transitory.

Nursing's product has always been hard to predict and evaluate. Our strained attempts to develop standards of care and quality assurance measures attest to this problem. Too often, we must resort to process variables based on surmise, rather than outcome variables based on fact. This persistent difficulty prompts the questions: What stimulates and sustains the service impulse, what creates the sense of social significance, when the results are so elusive? What can be held on to? What can be pointed to? And, even when results can be pointed to, how can isolated events, perceived as having meaning only for the individuals involved, be gathered into a giant configuration of nursing's aggregate impact? For how else could our place in public esteem and policymaking be earned and granted?

In the time of Florence Nightingale, the social significance of nursing, although perhaps narrowly focused on one individual, may have been at its zenith. The four essential elements mentioned earlier were all present. Miss Nightingale's sense of social purpose was sufficient to override the objections of her upper-class parents and the mores of her society when she entered nursing. Her well-placed confidence in her own capacities was unflagging. Her vision for nursing was vivid and far-reaching, and it was buttressed with instrumental detail. But perhaps most pertinent for this discussion of "product" is that she moved into a veritable wasteland of health care and thus was able to bring immediate and dramatic results that captured the attention and gratitude of the times. The nursing effort she organized during the Crimean War was responsible for lowering the death rate among the nation's fallen sons and warriors from 42 to 2.2 percent (2:42). Simple, striking data! Lives saved!

Furthermore, our professional forebear was politically astute enough that, when she returned to England, she capitalized on the credit earned on the battlefields of Scutari to force major structural and policy reforms in the health care system at home. Miss Nightingale's organizational acumen was felicitously joined to her zeal for the systematic investigation of health and environmental phenomena. For this, she has become known as "the passionate statistician." Indeed, she had something to point to.

How do we regain the vitalizing sense of purpose and sanction that existed in these origins of modern nursing? As has been said: education, research, and an impressive presence in the public eye, some of which will be discussed in later chapters.

But, for now, the recognition that an attitude of social significance is requisite for actualization as professionals suffices.

In self-searching fashion we might ask ourselves: Am I motivated to serve? Do I have confidence in my capacity to do so? Am I convinced that nursing is a significant force for social progress? Can I say specifically what is nursing's actual and potential contribution to society?

Our answers are a measure of our sense of social significance. Knowing this, we can proceed to consider how these convictions are translated into professional performance.

15

ULTIMACY OF PROFESSIONAL PERFORMANCE

"I have produced my works with as much care as I could" (4:4).

Thus Sartre defined *ultimacy* in his personal epitaph.

As was posited in the preceding chapter, our sense of social significance is founded on the alpha and the omega of our proposed nursing ideology: "I believe in nursing as an occupational force for social good . . ." and "I believe in myself . . . my responsibilities . . . my rights" (page 61). *Social significance* establishes the merit of our mission, as a profession, and our confidence in having a meritorious place, as an individual, in that mission. *Ultimacy of professional performance,* the quality of being ultimate or utmost, responds to significance as a moral imperative and pours this significance into the work itself. The voice of ultimacy reasons that, since nursing has great importance and we have cast our lot with the profession, we are obligated to give our *utmost* and do our *best.* Thus, it incorporates and combines quantitative and qualitative mandates regarding our nursing activities. Within the Becker and Carper elements of work identification among occupational environments, ultimacy would be the most profound degree of "commitment to task" (page 28).

In a profession proclaimed, as nursing has been described

in our beliefs, to be scientific, clinical, humanistic, and deserving of its maximum impact, *ultimacy* encompasses and commands all of the following concepts:

creativity
  science
    art
      technology

intellectual skill
technical skill
social skill

craftsmanship
expertise
excellence

assertiveness
  advocacy
    accountability
      autonomy
    activism

commitment
responsibility
leadership
perseverance
risk-taking
objectivity
integrity

legitimate power
legitimate control
legitimate authority

self-motivation
self-development
self-care
self-determination
self-governance

Ultimacy goes beyond each and defines the legitimacy and relationship of all; that is, ALL ARE NEEDED TO THE EXTENT THAT THEY STRIVE TOWARD THE ULTIMATE IN PROFESSIONAL PERFORMANCE.

Ultimacy, as an attitude, carefully avoids the perils and poisons of perfectionism—that is, unrealistic goals, unreasonable demands, an eventually faltering spirit. Where ultimacy motivates, the most and the best are good enough.

Ultimacy, as an intense driving force, requires collegiality to balance it out. As nurses striving for our personal best, we need to serve as true colleagues to one another to augment our individual performance, as well as to offer support, perspective, and validation to each other.

Whether viewed from an individual or collective standpoint, *ultimacy* is not principally directed toward external competition or status. ULTIMACY does NOT fundamentally seek SUPREMACY. UTMOST does NOT necessarily mean UPPERMOST. However, higher rank may be a means to or a by-product of ultimacy, or both. That is, superordinacy may, on occasion, be necessary for nursing to be heard or felt, and/or it may be accorded by society for a job well done and well appreciated. But ultimacy is not essentially a race against another individual or discipline. Each reaches for hers/its best; but, most effectively, we reach together.

To put this within the framework of the nursing universe proposed earlier, *ultimacy*, issuing from a moral imperative for nursing, demands: the fullest development of the discipline and practice; the fullest development of the individual in that discipline and practice; and the fullest development of the social context for the nurse and the profession to act on and within most beneficially.

NURSING UNIVERSE

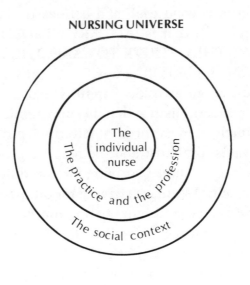

Stated another way:

Ultimacy requires that

> The nurse be as well-prepared in knowledge, skill, and attitude as she can be and perform to the utmost of her ability.
>
> The science, art, and technology of the practice constantly advance.
>
> The settings for education and practice and the policies, structures, and resources that influence them enhance the effect of the nurse and the practice on the client.

Ultimacy leads to

> The best outcome for the client achievable, as the above requirements are met.

Ultimacy can be seen in every arena of nursing practice. Ultimacy is seen in knowledgeable, creative, sensitive caring for patients; teaching of students; and management of groups and systems. It is seen in the meticulous construction of the scientific base for all nursing practice. It is seen in the skillful consensus-building within the contorted channels and among the heterogeneous interests comprising organized nursing. It is seen in the adroit maneuvering of nursing practice act amendments through the treacherous vicissitudes of state legislative process. It is seen in gaining coveted seats at social policy tables and in performing admirably in those positions.

It is possible to talk with some fluency and certainty about what ultimacy leads to. But what leads to ultimacy is another, not-so-easy matter. Frequent, universal complaints are: "People just don't take pride in their work any more." And "What happened to craftsmanship?" In nursing, these grumbles translate into: "Nurses don't nurse; they don't care." "Nurses won't work nights and weekends." There are references to "appliance" nurses, who just put in their time and then only when they need the money for a new refrigerator.

What leads to a sense of 24-hour, 365-day, year-after-year commitment to and accountability for one's major work?

While one cannot discount the attitudes brought by students to their nursing programs from eighteen or more years of social conditioning, the educational climate in nursing schools is a major factor in the development of professional qualities. Somewhere in the interaction between the socializers and the socializees—that is, between the faculty and clinical role models and the students—it is essential that the attitude of ultimacy be engendered and nurtured. An important influence within this concentrated environment is the way teachers are seen to approach their own work and how they guide and evaluate the learner in his. Where ultimacy is valued, standards of performance will fix their attention on the now-and-future "patient"-client just as firmly as on the immediate student-client. This is not to suggest that there is no margin for error, but rather that there is no margin for indifference nor for persistent falling short. Students are first exposed to the standards of the profession through the standards set for them as learners. While this is not a complete and lasting experience in ultimacy, it is a critical beginning.

Although all of us in nursing are entrusted with socializing our professional progeny, teachers of nursing play a major role in this responsibility. Our own sense of ultimacy demands that we strive to the best of our ability to instill ultimacy in others. But obstacles present themselves. Ultimacy is an attitude. Attitudes are hard to teach and they are hard to evaluate. Pressures are on us as faculty (1) to ignore that which cannot be objectively measured, lest we open ourselves to charges of discrimination, and (2) to respect other people's values and attitudes whether we agree with them or not. We must weigh these pressures against our commitment to ultimacy in ourselves and in those admitted to the profession. Our carefully developed, internally calibrated, professional judgment is not a vice to disclaim and arrest but a subjective tool to prize and put to good purpose in guiding the educational process. We are not just purveyors and employers, but instruments as well, in the indoctrination of newcomers to the field.

What does all of this mean in practical terms? How does this attitude of ultimacy come into play in our lives as nurses? How can we be "as well-prepared in knowledge, skill, and attitude" as we can be and "perform to the utmost of this ability"?

As a beginning, we might refer to those concepts bound up within ultimacy and listed on page 129. In a nutshell, they propose that we take charge of our professional selves; that, in a deliberate way, we participate in the advancement of nursing science and practice; that we maintain ourselves in mind and spirit at the forefront of that practice; and that we accept no impediments to the fullest use of our talents.

First and foremost, ultimacy requires a career plan rather than a job orientation. When the former prevails, we conceive of work experiences as a progression, even though they may be interrupted or part-time. Decisions about employment and education are not made purely in terms of immediate payoffs but in terms of long-range goals. We constantly negotiate adjustments between our personal and professional lives so that our professional selves can grow and mature. As we peer at ourselves in our professional mirror, we do not want to discover a Dorian Grey–like image, frozen in our graduation uniforms, static on the surface, crumbling within. We want to see ourselves take on the look of curiosity, seasoned sagacity, stature, and satisfaction—the look of self-actualization.

Maintaining a career attitude is particularly difficult in nursing's present environment. In reviewing the literature in Section Two, we came to recognize the authority, accountability, and advancement problems created when professions are practiced within organizations. In this regard, nursing has suffered more than most emerging professions because, in addition to being a women's field, we labor under a cruel historical circumstance. In this country, graduate nurses, who had been independently employed in homes while students and "untrained" nurses staffed the hospitals, were first driven into institutions for a livelihood during the depths of the depression of the 1930s. Thus, they were at the mercy of their employers, powerless to bargain for the working conditions appropriate to their training and service. We have never fully recovered from this adverse beginning. Work settings have not provided career paths. Except for isolated successes, a hierarchy of clinical competence has not materialized in roles, authority, or compensation.

Changes in ourselves must be matched with changes in health care agencies and even in the larger social picture. The organization and policies of health care systems must respect and reward the progressive expertise we are determined to achieve and practice. And society must come to appreciate, expect, and pay for the benefits of continuous, expert caring as opposed to a melange of hands and feet. *Thus, ultimacy causes us to recognize that, beyond growth in ourselves and the improvement of practice, we bear the responsibility to stimulate contextual reform.* This requires that many of us include in our professional armamentaria understanding and skill in conflict resolution, organizational theory, economics, change theory, power, and politics.

However, organizational and political acumen alone will not suffice because, in addition to being frustrated by forces and constraints in and around the practice environment, we are drained or "burned out" by the task itself. By intimate, intense, sustained contact with patients and their troubles. By the hassles associated in getting a nursing unit to function properly. By the competing demands of a teaching position. By the numerous stresses to which students are subjected. Because of these difficulties in the job itself, *ultimacy dictates that, in the midst of these immediate, crushing responsibilities, we maintain an objective long-range perspective, that we seek and cherish personal support systems, and that we periodically pull back for refreshment and objectivity to assure forward movement.*

In sum, ultimacy demands that we keep a hand on the controls of our professional lives; that we neither stand still in our professional development, nor be swept along in the environmental currents; and that we not allow ourselves to spin dizzily within the intensity of the immediate task until we are exhausted and defeated. Rather, ultimacy requires that we progress in a purposeful way toward our individual best as nurses and the collective best of nursing.

In self-appraisal we might ask: Do I have career goals? Do I have a plan for gaining the experience and education to achieve them? What particular knowledge and skill and what personal qualities do I need to develop to be most effective in practice? What support systems have I established? What special contribution do I intend to make to the science and technology of nursing—that is, what shall I add to the middle ring of the nursing universe that will transcend and endure beyond my presence? What can I point to as a reflection of the ultimacy of my performance?

Now to consider how we join our ultimacy with that of others who share our unique social significance to achieve our individual and corporate destinies.

16

COLLEGIALITY AND COLLECTIVITY

I believe in myself *and in my nursing colleagues* . . .

I believe that nursing's maximum contribution for social betterment is dependent on . . . the ability of the profession to maintain *unity* within diversity.

On collegiality and collectivity, from the "Declaration of Belief," p. 61

Although we may not find the analogy appealing, there is a lot to be learned about collegiality and collectivity from a football game:

From the team—in which the members realize that they must work together to reach their goal; that the success of one in his role depends on the success of others in theirs

From the bleachers—where the swells of an enormously powerful support system emerge when synchrony is applied to noisy enthusiasm

Collegiality and collectivity are two concepts from the large collection of "co-" words: coalition, cooperation, collaboration, coherence, cohesion, compact, community, and others. All, with subtle differences, extend the meaning of their prefix, connoting "with, together, joint." From among them, I have chosen this particular pair for their complementarity and comprehensiveness. *Collegiality,* meaning shared responsibility and authority, has to do with the micro, dyadic level in nursing. *Collectivity,* the quality of wholeness, of being one body, has to do with the macro, corporate level. Just as these words stem from the same root, they signify variations of the same fundamental attitude. Therefore, their separation for our discussion is somewhat of a contrived, conceptual, and analytical convenience.

In combination, collegiality and collectivity recall a resounding theme in the writings on professions. Such terms as

> brotherhood/sisterhood
> control by peers
> colleague esteem
> mutual support
> professional affiliation
> collective autonomy

appear repeatedly.

Collectivity

I pledged in an earlier chapter that since our freedom is such a "heartfelt issue" with us, space would be set aside for its consideration. I hasten to do so here in introducing the subject of collectivity, lest you immediately turn a blind eye to the page. Some persons, particularly those in aspiring professions and some naturally free spirits, may see independence and collectivity as inherently antagonistic to one another.

As a suppressed, if not actually oppressed, occupation, buffeted by hegemonic forces and undervalued politically, socially, and economically, we evidence a natural preoccupation with freedom, independence, autonomy, control, power, and high places. Yet, in many of our acts of commission and omission, we deny our own access to these talismans. Gilb, quoted in the literature, points out the obvious paradox that so often escapes us:

> One of the paradoxes of American life is that when Americans talk about freedom for the individual, they generally band together into organizations to do it. Why does this paradox exist—for example, in the professions? Freedom in a complex, interdependent economy comes *through* organizations. Without an organization to define and sustain his areas of freedom, the average individual professional would often not be able to be free. (1:53)

I referred previously to nursing, enormous in its numbers and inestimable in its services, yet potentialized rather than actualized as a profession. We have been likened to a Sleeping Giant. Relating this imagery to the paradox above, it seems to me that, in responding to the cry for independence, we have progressed from total somnolence to jangling nerve endings and hyperkinesis, lacking the coordinated action necessary to achieve the freedom whose call aroused us.

Nursing's collective body is diverse indeed, ranging from practical nurses to postdoctoral fellows; from those who work with the well or with whole communities, industries, or schools, to those who tend the comatose bodies and the attached hardware of the critically ill; from those who manage patients to those who manage health care systems; and from generalists who circulate within those systems to specialists who restrict themselves to certain procedures or illnesses or ages.

Nursing subcultures and interest groups have sprung up and are becoming organized locally, regionally, nationally, and internationally. Nursing service administrators, to some extent reacting to or recoiling from the economic and general welfare emphasis of the American Nurses' Association, have split off into several different directions. Also, clinical interest organizations are developing rapidly in number and size. Some hold national meetings better attended than the ANA biennial conventions, and a new layer, a federation of specialty nursing organizations, has formed.

This proliferation of interest groups can well be understood against the backdrop of an increasingly complex and depersonalized society in which vocational interests have narrowed to preserve the individual's sense of identity. This phenomenon can also be understood as a means of developing and concentrating knowledge and expertise within a wide and intricate field. On the other hand, it complicates the processes for preserving wholeness and possesses the potential for dividing allegiances.

To assure that one forum is maintained for voices to be heard, decisions to be made, and action to be taken that concern our whole body and to rally identification with the total profession, it is axiomatic that nursing must maintain one all-embracing professional society. And, as a major expression of *our sense of collectivity, we are called to join and participate in that society,* as well as in other organizations that may appeal to and reflect our special interests. Not as a symbolic gesture toward professionalism, but as acknowledgment of the self-governance and power necessary for us to carry out our social contract. As Gilb reminds us, "to define and sustain . . . [our] freedom" (1:53).

In turn, it is self-evident that the professional society, currently the ANA, must reach out to us and, through its structure, programs, and resources, listen to, guide, assist, and be advocates for all of us within the profession. With its corporate might, our brotherhood/sisterhood should stand behind the nurse, who, in rightfully exercising her ultimacy, has to *push against* the constraints of the profession or the social context to *push out* the boundaries of practice.

In a splendid article on "Dilemmas of Democracy in the Voluntary Association," which is commendable reading, Robert Merton, a distinguished authority on the professions, has pointed out the need for such associations to hear all voices within them. "The democratic organization must provide for periodic audits of dissent as well as assent. . . . It thus provides occasion for dissent to modify the thinking of the majority" (3:1056). It follows that we must not allow our nursing society to silence minority voices, be they from disgruntled members or disdainful nonmembers, for dissatisfaction and discontent sharpen the cutting edge of change.

Coalition-building with other professional organizations and citizens' groups is an effective means of enlarging our influence. However, for nursing to be a full, rather than a token, participant in such arrangements, we must have a strong, cohesive, well-informed force to bring to the union. Too often we have allowed ourselves to be divided and swallowed up in a pretended partnership—for example, in joint certification and accreditation endeavors with other professions. Caution reminds us therefore that *internal collectivity precedes and enhances external coalescence.*

For those who fear suffocation, it should be explained that, as used here in the context of professionhood:

Collectivity does not
   stifle individual opinion

It does
   stimulate it
   collect it
   develop it
   enhance it
   challenge it
   balance it
   validate it

Collectivity does not discourage individual initiative	It does guide it augment it protect it appreciate it
Collectivity does not deny individual responsibility and accountability	It does demand it organize it evaluate it

Collectivity is not the attitude underlying "groupiness" behavior, but that which might better be called "groupness." *Groupiness*, to my mind, connotes a group-think, molasses-like lethargy, suppression of stellarism, denial of expert authority, unrealistic egalitarianism, oppressive togetherness mentality, which strives for the lowest common denominator in every situation. Conversely, *groupness* describes those behaviors resulting from a true, not misguided, sense of collectivity—those behaviors that "define and sustain the individual's area of freedom" and augment his powers.

Collectivity, however, does dilute extremism and retard radical change. This aspect of collectivity will be viewed with favor or disfavor, depending on where one stands on the particular issue at stake. For sure, it frustrates the radicalizers. But overall, it must be seen as an advantage, because it prevents the destructive effects of anarchy and the energy drain and loss of progression caused by wild swings of the pendulum.

Collegiality

First, with feeling. The ideology speaks of the humanity of the nurse engaging the humanity of the client. This may be easier to achieve than the extension of our humanity into that of our associates. Nursing has yet to develop a strong professional ethos that instills deeply within each of us a camaraderie not easily shaken by jealousies, disagreements, defection, and even ennui. This, I believe, is a characteristic of physicians that we should admire, study, and emulate.

To refer again to the two concentric rings of the self-concept (page 106), collegiality is the actual sharing of that innermost core identity with our colleagues, a spiritual brotherhood or sisterhood. True professionhood, *perhaps above all else,* means that we are as bonded to our associates—through conviction and calling, through social contract, through professional thought and conscience—as we are bonded to our natural sisters through blood. Professionhood means that the I-Nursing relationship envelops us all in a common cause. This professional bond causes pride when a colleague triumphs and pain when she fails. It causes a loyalty that does not blind us to her faults but opens our eyes to her virtues. It causes us to confront her in disagreement, disappointment, and disapproval and to stand beside her in determination.

Collegiality is as sacred as a vow; it is a solemn promise whereby we bind ourselves to those who share our cause, our convictions, our identity, our destiny.

Now, with dispassion. Collegiality, the sharing of responsibility and authority with our colleagues, is an attitude about our individual nurse-to-nurse relationships. It is based on ultimacy and leads to respect. The first recognizes that doing nursing's work to the utmost is enhanced by an appropriate collaborative effort; recognizes that, through genuine collaboration, individual endeavor is potentiated, not just pooled. Respect then follows, with the acknowledgment and encouragement of the contribution that others make to our mutual task.

In addition to its instrumental function in magnifying individual accomplishment, collegiality serves a vital expressive function. It cools the flames of misfired ultimacy that often result in reality shock in the neophyte nurse and in burnout in the veteran practitioner or faculty member. Collegiality lends company, assistance, and added perspective to those situations in which unrealistic expectations, a feeling of alienation, and loss of humanity threaten to take over.

Collegiality presents a special challenge in that it involves a delicate balance as signaled in the aforementioned adjectives, "appropriate" and "genuine." Comprehending and practicing collegiality requires that we be conscious of the extremes and the middle ground in relation to both the *responsibility* and *authority* that are our joint properties with our associates. For a moment, let us touch on the tensions within both aspects of this common ground.

The extreme attitudes relative to *responsibility* are those of abdication and monopoly. Collegiality advocates neither. Abdication of responsibility is a contradiction in terms; it is, by definition, irresponsible. As to monopoly, in a job as big as ours, there is more than enough responsibility for all. Individually borne, it is unrealistic and intolerable. Collectively borne, it is hardly bearable. In the sensitive equipoise between the "I am responsible" and "they are responsible" is the "we are responsible" attitude, which carries with it the awareness that we do not have to solve all of the problems of the world single-handedly. It carries the trust that others will take over where we leave off, when we have done our best. It carries the realization that elements of primary and secondary responsibility may operate in every situation, rotating among us as time and circumstance require.

In the realm of *authority*, the balance is largely between

the positional and expert forms, whether in a nursing education or practice setting. Collegiality urges us to defer to expert
authority in professional matters and to hierarchal authority,
if it is not 'the same, in administrative matters. Where these
clash, the value of communication and compromise, two
tools of collegiality, becomes apparent, and the techniques of
conflict resolution may come into play. The greatest wisdom
is in distinguishing between principles that cannot be sac-
rificed and differences in style or opinion or short-term disagreements that may be less important in the final outcome.
Ultimacy should be the meeting place where both types of
authority are negotiated and reconciled. Thus, the question,
"What is essential for achieving the utmost in performance?"
is the critical one for sorting out the issues.

In a very practical sense, how should we relate to one another as colleagues and collaborators in the nursing enterprise? Guidelines can be recited staccato fashion, proving that
difficulty is in the behaving and not the knowing. However, it
is good to keep in mind that collegiality:

- Deemphasizes status differences in responsibility and authority; the task organizes the work; leadership and followship
fluctuate

- Focuses on the functional, rather than dysfunctional, aspects of
individual performance; accepts foibles

- Promotes sharing of information, recognizing this as necessary
for task accomplishment as well as for individual growth; this
ranges from personal reporting on one level to scholarly
communication through professional journals on another

- Takes seriously the opinions of others; hears dissent objectively

- Takes seriously the work of others and builds on it

- Values peer review and both offers and receives constructive criticism

- Encourages risk-taking in ourselves and others by joint problem-solving and mutual support

- Stresses remediation, rather than blame-setting or blame avoidance

And others you could add to this catechism of collegiality.

Where are such behaviors first learned? What conditions in the educational environment foster collectivity? Schools traditionally place a high value on independent effort. In fact, collaboration, in some situations, is called cheating, and grading is competitive in most instances. Despite this general attitude, students, sometimes with faculty encouragement, cluster in support groups, study groups, special interest groups, protest groups, and others. Additional opportunities for experiencing collegiality are group projects—most effectively combining faculty and students—clinical conferences, and observations of the collective efforts of teachers and other professional role models.

The point of transition from education into practice is unquestionably another critical period in the socialization of nursing progeny. We all bear a heavy responsibility for welcoming them into our professional community by displaying all of the behaviors outlined earlier. Chapter 20 amplifies this process.

The literature review pointed to the effects of organizations on professional collegiality. Institutional values, structures, and processes may facilitate or impede this attitude and behavior. Problems associated with this institutional-professional relationship are evident in health care agencies and academia as well.

As to hospitals, from my vantage point, it seems that the concept of shared responsibility and authority is inherent in primary nursing in which colleagues serve as associate nurses. Of course, collegiality may also be fostered in other types of staffing patterns, but it may be less assured. When organizations resist nurse collegiality by insisting on accountability and responsibility only through pyramidal arrangements that lead to non-nurses not qualified to set and judge standards for nursing, major reforms must be effected. On the other hand, in unionized facilities where nurses do occupy hierarchal positions, collegiality may be seriously strained as nurses oppose each other at the bargaining tables. Professional governance within health care organizations is an area deserving of much attention and development. The preservation of collegiality demands it.

Within educational settings, faculties of nursing have seemed to cycle through team and independent teaching, as they initially welcomed the camaraderie and stimulation of working together and then came to feel oppressed by the closeness and depleted by the time consumed in the process. Integrated curricula, which swallowed huge chunks of content, demand teaming by overtaxing the special knowledge and capacities of individuals. Today maintaining the equilibrium between individual and collaborative effort in academia is especially difficult but essential for maximum achievement in times of scarce resources.

Students, faculty, administrators, and practitioners alike confront the same persistent questions. What socialization methods and organizational arrangements encourage and enable the spirit of *collegiality*? As we formulate the answers, our sense of *social significance* and *ultimacy* stirs us to find ways to implement these solutions and, assuredly, *collectivity* will be necessary to achieve them.

————

Final food for thought: is the true meaning of collegiality and collectivity that each of us becomes all of us?

————

17

THE THREESOME

Although each of the qualities for professionhood described in the preceding essays is of critical importance, their
mutuality and totality are equally important. Together, these
qualities are essential to activate and energize the nursing
ideology declared in Section Three.

By the definitions given:

Social significance is certainty about the nature and importance of our work. It is the sense of mission and social sanction.

Ultimacy is commitment to doing our most and our best in
our work.

Collegiality and collectivity are the conviction that responsibility and authority are shared and that the wholeness of the
profession must be preserved.

Translated into personal litanies, these attitudes remind
us, respectively, that:

Nursing has great social importance.

Therefore, I must perform to the best of my ability.

Nursing is most effective as a collaborative and collective
effort.

The values underlying these attitudes are, respectively:

Health

Individual effort

Unity

Each of these qualities has both individual and collective dimensions:

Social significance embodies individual belief in the overall worth of nursing and in the particular worth of one's own work.

Launched from this sense of manifest purpose, *ultimacy* impels us to perform the work to its greatest possible attainment; individual works mounting up to the grand accomplishments and the corporate social impact of the profession.

Through *collectivity* and *collegiality,* the professional agenda takes shape and is advanced; individual efforts are given general direction and perspective and support and magnification.

Each attribute is critical; each enhances its companions; no two can stand without the third:

Ultimacy and collectivity, without social significance, have no purpose.

Social significance and collectivity, without ultimacy, lose the substance of the effort; they are purpose and process without content, without task accomplishment.

Social significance and ultimacy, without collectivity, are isolated, unstable, and enfeebled.

In combination, these cardinal virtues lead to the good of society, the good of the profession, the good of each of us.

When all this is believed, the principal objective of the socialization process in nursing must be the incorporation of the attitudes of social significance, ultimacy, and collegiality/collectivity within each of us. This realization guides us to the setting where these qualities should take root—to nursing education, our next subject for discussion.

REFERENCE LIST FOR SECTION FIVE

1. Gilb, C. *Hidden hierarchies: The professions and government.* New York: Harper & Row, 1966.
2. Kalisch, P.A., & Kalisch, B.J. *The advance of American nursing.* Boston: Little, Brown, & Co., 1978.
3. Merton, R.K. Dilemmas of democracy in the voluntary association. *American Journal of Nursing,* 1960, *66,* 1055-1061.
4. Sartre, J.-P. Author-philosopher Sartre dies. In *San Francisco Chronicle,* April 16, 1980, p. 4. Quoted from one of Sartre's final statements published in mid-March in *Le Nouvel Observateur.*

THE FOUNDATIONS OF NURSING PRACTICE

A BIBLICAL FABLE ON OUR ORIGINS

In the beginning, God created nursing.

He (or She) said, I will take a solid, simple, significant system of *education* and an adequate, applicable base of clinical *research*, and

On these rocks, will I build My greatest gift to Mankind—nursing practice.

On the seventh day, He——threw up His hands.

And has left it up to us.

I believe in nursing as a professional discipline, requiring a sound education and research base grounded in its own science and in the variety of academic and professional disciplines with which it relates.

From the Declaration of Belief About the Nature and Purpose of Nursing (page 61)

18

NURSING EDUCATION

A troubled past

Nursing education: the major *raison d'être* for much of my professional life. Hence it is realistic to expect greater intensity in this chapter, particularly where pet peeves are concerned. In fact, in whatever stage of our careers, objectivity is difficult for all of us to achieve in reviewing the nursing education scene and drawing up a blueprint for the future. We carry our nursing school experiences around with us like childhood scars that our fingers worry over endlessly. So reminded, we tend to behave like parents—some determined that their offspring be exposed to the same upbringing as themselves, others insisting on quite another treatment for those who follow in their footsteps. We may stand a better chance of escaping our personal histories and developing a more creative attitude if we begin by stepping back from the inner circles of the nursing universe and looking, through the literature, at the broader field of professional education.

PROFESSIONAL EDUCATION IN GENERAL

The readings on professionalization in Section Two provide a backdrop of historical context, as well as modern day concern about professional education, against which to examine nursing's development.

One of the essentials of the professionalization of an occupation is the forming of close ties with academia. On this requirement, Parsons was perhaps most emphatic in asserting that the institutionalization of the professional discipline in the universities lies at the core of the professional system (21:536ff). This close profession-university alignment has had significant implications for the image and status of professions, the admission and indoctrination of aspirants to the field, the creation of the knowledge base for practice, and the values espoused. As a consequence, a number of questions and challenges have arisen about education for the professions today. I have attempted to summarize these below from the readings and from my professional experience:

1. Whom does the professional school serve? Who is/are the client(s) in a complex system involving the profession, faculty, students, practitioners, institutions, consumers?

2. Are professionals prepared for practice in a changing world of diverse clients?

3. How are students socialized into the values and norms of the profession?

4. Does the school set appropriate standards for the profession through its selection, instructional, and evaluation processes?

5. Does the school have an ongoing influence on practitioners?

6. What is the actual/ideal effect of academia on reform in the profession?

157

7. Does self-actualization, or work satisfaction, occur? For the faculty? For the student? For the practicing nurse?

8. Are the values of the basic disciplines and the profession compatible? What tensions exist between the two within academia?

9. Are the values of the academic and the practice branches of the profession compatible? What intraprofessional tensions exist between the two?

10. Are the research efforts dedicated to improving the quality of life?

It should be noted that the crux of these concerns is the relationship of education to practice or, more bluntly, the effects of the separation between the two. And serving to compound the education——practice division within professions is another schism now widening in the universities: the schism between the professional and the academic disciplines. This latter cleavage was less troublesome in the halcyon days of university expansion. During the current retrenchment phase, however, when there is competition for students and resources, a backlash has occurred against the professional schools, which draw more of both. We, in the professions, are accused by our basic arts and science counterparts of being too expensive, too independent, too specialized, and too self-serving. Some "pure academicians" would go so far as to suggest that undergraduate professional programs be "taught in independent technical schools or condensed in intensive graduate programs" conducted separately from the university's graduate school (15:48). (Were such a proposition to gain popularity, nursing might find itself in isolation once again.)

The ten questions posed earlier in the chapter are good ones for professional schools to ask of themselves and of more impartial judges, as they engage in periodic self-examination. And we should bear them in mind as we proceed to consider nursing education: What has happened and what should happen?

NURSING EDUCATION IN PARTICULAR

Nursing is faithfully acting out the scenario for the struggling professions, but in its own inimitable way. It is true that: (1) We have been moving into the universities, setting up autonomy for education and a dichotomy between the academic and practice branches. (2) We are attempting a grudging mix of academic and service values. (3) We are either fussing with or striking up uneasy friendships with our fellows in the opposite branch. (4) We are bent on constructing the knowledge base underlying nursing practice. In respect to each of these developments, nursing has added its special topography to the landscape of professional environments.

Entering the higher education mainstreams

(One toe at a time.) Yes, we have been moving into the academic establishment in a most halting, confusing, self-defeating manner. Consider these current levels of preparation and credentials for *entry* into the nursing field:

- Nursing assistant: short-term, on-the-job training; institutional certificate, if any credential
- Practical/vocational nurse: postsecondary education of approximately one year; institutional diploma; practical/vocational license

159

- Registered nurse: postsecondary education of two to three years under hospital auspices; hospital diploma; "professional" license

- Registered nurse: postsecondary education of two years usually under community college auspices; associate degree in nursing; "professional" license

- Registered nurse: postsecondary education of four years under college or university auspices; baccalaureate degree in nursing; "professional" license

- Registered nurse: postbaccalaureate education of three years under university auspices; master's degree in nursing (M.N.); "professional" license

- And, our 1979 registered nurse addition: postbaccalaureate education of three years under university auspices; doctoral degree in nursing (N.D.); "professional" license

Consider, too, these positions on education for nursing practice:

- Florence Nightingale proposed that nursing schools be financially independent of any service institutions with which they are affiliated. (10:989)

- Esther Lucile Brown's 1948 revered exposition for the Russell Sage Foundation, *Nursing for the Future*, proposed that the term "professional" be restricted to those nurses who graduated from university or university-affiliated programs. (8)

- The American Nurses' Association 1965 position paper advocating
  - That all nursing education be in institutions of higher learning.
  - That there be two levels of nursing practice: professional, for which baccalaureate education in nursing would be the minimum preparation; and technical, for which associate degree education in nursing would be the minimum preparation. (1)

□ The ANA's 1978 resolutions on "entry into practice" mandating

  • Two categories of nursing practice by 1985: the professional, requiring baccalaureate preparation, with distinct title, credential, and competencies to be determined; and an unnamed category, requiring associate degree preparation, with distinct title, credential, and competencies to be determined.

  • The development of a mechanism for deriving competency statements for the two categories of practice, by 1980.

  • Opportunities for educational mobility to facilitate movement from the yet untitled category to the professional. (3:9)

And, finally, consider that, as the 1980s unfurl:

□ In the United States, there are 1389 programs preparing for R.N. licensure alone. Of these, 333 are hospital diploma; 688 are associate degree; 368 are generic (prelicensure) baccalaureate programs (20:82); two generic master's; and one generic doctoral program.

□ In 1978 there were 1329 programs preparing for L.V.N./ L.P.N. licensure. (19:113)

□ There are 958,308 R.N.'s employed in nursing; 722,861 (75.4 percent) hold less than a baccalaureate as their highest academic credential, 158,086 (16.5 percent) the baccalaureate in nursing, 31,262 (3.3 percent) the baccalaureate in other fields, 26,608 (2.8 percent) the master's degree in nursing, 13,162 (1.4 percent) the master's in other fields, 1,846 (0.2 percent) the doctorate, and 4,483 (0.5 percent) not reporting educational preparation. (2:14)

□ No state yet requires baccalaureate education in nursing for professional licensure and practice.

□ Statements of competencies for the newly defined professional nurse are still in process. (4:13)

□ Hiring policies seldom discriminate between the baccalaureate and the associate degree and diploma nurses.

The first list of considerations—those SEVEN! entry
points into nursing practice—attests to nursing's tendency
toward infinite accommodation, a quality deliberately excluded from those recommended for professionhood in Section Five. We have woven a tangled web by adding more and
more layers to our struggling frame, without shedding former
modes. Thus, we have given credence to the nurse-is-a-nurse
image; confounded ourselves; confounded the public; diffused
and dissipated accountability; undermined salary structures;
and put ourselves in a weak position for collaborating with
other health professionals.

The second list of considerations—a chronology of policy
statements—attests to expert and authoritative efforts to ar-
ticulate clear directions for the profession in education and
credentialing. The third list—recent data on programs, graduates, licensing, and remuneration—attests to our progress in
moving toward these established objectives. Viewed in this
fashion, it is apparent that the web results, not so much from
official indecision within nursing (because these hard-fought
battles have been waged and decided within our professional
society, the ANA), but more from grass roots reluctance and
resistance, aided and abetted by external forces. Such forces as
organized medicine and hospital administration have been
prone to see our upgrading efforts as potentially upsetting to
the sensitive economic and power bases in the health field and
have been blinded to the potential cost-effective health care
benefits. A heightened sense of collectivity, as well as an
awareness of the effects of these internal and external factions
on our services and our personal fortunes, would enable us to
make a giant leap forward toward the establishment of a

"solid, simple, significant" system of nursing education, as the fable foretold (page 154).

It must also be recognized that, as rival to both the existing multilevel happenstance and the two-tiered pattern proposed and repeatedly confirmed by the ANA, there is a minority opinion that *all* nursing education be at the baccalaureate or higher level. One group of this persuasion is the Association of Operating Room Nurses (5). Advocates of this position see this as the only way of achieving professionalism for nursing and commensurate status for its practitioners. Around no other single issue are the lines between the traditionalizers and professionalizers (page 103) so plainly drawn. Yet, ironically, both are fundamentally conservative positions. While one seeks to preserve the traditions of our past in nursing education, the other seeks to preserve the traditions of academia and the professionalism ideal.

Where would adherence to the beliefs declared in Section Three put us in this controversy? In the first place, the emphasis on "the ability of the profession to maintain unity" would support the right and the responsibility of our professional society, with our participation, to promulgate our official position. On that basis alone, the ideology would make us advocates of the ANA proposals.

On an even more fundamental plane, Beliefs II, III, and IV describe nursing as science, technology, and humanism in its development and its practice. (In respect to these first two dimensions, Esther Lucile Brown likened nursing to the engineering profession [8:143].) Thus, it seems a logical conclusion that such a broad field encompass two essential levels of practice and education. Otherwise, all who engage in the most repetitious, standardized nursing functions must, too, be advanced clinical scientists, or we must accept the equally untenable alternative of giving up either the science or the technology to another field.*

If we agree that the same preparation is not required of the advanced clinical scientists and their technical associates then we confront the question of where, within the system of higher education in this country, these two levels best fit. In my opinion, there is evidence that, whether or not we like their current methods and results, associate degree programs have been appropriately conceived to prepare humanistic technologists in nursing. The scientists and advanced clinicians, needed to work in tandem with the nurse technician to develop and apply the knowledge base for nursing and to practice, manage, and teach in complex nursing settings, must be both liberally and professionally educated to a much greater degree. The baccalaureate must be seen as only a beginning for these purposes and may very shortly be judged inadequate to fulfill the increasing demands of professional practice; this would require that the base be raised to graduate level. The daring move at Case Western Reserve University to establish the first generic (pre-licensure) doctoral program in nursing (N.D.) provides us with an opportunity to observe what dimensions will thereby be added to nursing and to nurses.

The associate nurse and the clinical scientist must work side by side, both with excellence, both committed to ulti-

---

*Please let us not permit these words to act as barriers between us. *Advanced clinical science* and *technology* are used here in a generic, not a naming sense. The profession has long found that no terms are ideal for our purposes. However, *technology* and *technologist* convey an educational level of common understanding; technology refers to providing the means necessary for human sustenance and comfort. The humanistic aspect of nursing, in my view, is bound up in both the clinical science and the technology.

macy of performance. And both must be respected. However, to avoid the existing problems of our entangling web, identity and accountability must be exquisitely clear to the public in the future—through titles, licenses, positions, authority, performance, and, not insignificantly, remuneration. Also, to give rationality to our growth, the question of relative numbers of nurses needed in the two categories to achieve the greatest good should continue to be addressed. The Western Interstate Commission for Higher Education for Nursing (WICHE) manpower project, *Nursing Resources and Requirements: A Guide for State-Level Planning*, has made a significant step in this direction by presenting a new way to project nursing requirements and the resources necessary to meet those needs within states (13).

Influences and effects within academia

Setting aside now this exhausting tracing of nursing's faltering zigzag courses *into* academia, we could concentrate on nursing's adventures *within* the hallowed halls of higher learning. It would be of interest to consider (1) the influence that particular *affiliations* have had on our development; (2) the stresses of *conflicting roles and values;* (3) the effects of the *separation from nursing service;* and (4) specialized *accreditation* as a potent force in our history.

We could begin soon after the turn of this century with our first academic ties. Our early nursing leaders, seeking university degrees to enhance their capabilities and credibility, found schools of education to be most hospitable. So we first took up with the educationists who, although elite in their discipline that grew out of (or outgrew) the normal school tradition, were of marginal respectability in the university. They seemed happy for our companionship, as newcomers, also in a helping field even lower in the pecking order. Nurses studied the procedures, methods, and processes of elementary, secondary, and higher education and brought them back to be assimilated within the practice, values, and language of nursing. Hence, pedagogy has become part of our basic heritage.

Then with the advent of the federally funded Nurse Scientist program of the 1960s and 1970s, nurses were encouraged to go into the social and, later, with some trepidation, the natural sciences. And those disciplines, some with declining enrollments, gladly received them and the accompanying institutional subsidies. With this impetus and the growth of doctoral programs in nursing, the range of doctorates earned by nurse faculty has broadened.

It will be interesting to observe the long-range impact of this line of affiliation on the profession. Or, to be retrospective in a moment of idle speculation, we might turn the clock back seventy-five years to the early part of the century. Imagine twenty ambitious nurses, destined to be leaders, enrolled for graduate study in departments of physics, biochemistry, physiology, and microbiology, and rewrite the history of nursing to the present. A fascinating epic would unfold.

As a corollary to our developing partnership with these basic and applied disciplines, albeit not without ambivalence, we have been disengaging philosophically and structurally from the profession of medicine, a natural alliance. Why? Undoubtedly because patronage was their best offer when what we needed, earned, insisted on, and were receiving from others was collegiality.

Overall, it can be seen that *our values, our practice, and our research all reflect the company we have kept in this progression through the academy.*

Next, to further explain nursing's peculiar variation on the theme of professional education, we could consider the degree and effect of the gap between schooling and service. For several decades, nursing education has, by and large, gone its separate way from the practice branch. Even hospital diploma programs in recent years have been significantly immunized against the demands of the service environs. Collegiate programs have worked mightily to assume the characteristics of academia and to take on full rank and privilege within their parent institutions of higher learning. Faculty credentials are increasingly impressive. Nurses participate actively in the broad processes of academic governance. Federal grants have given us independent means and the envious respect of peers in other disciplines. Admissions standards have risen overall, although to some extent they continue to fluctuate with the size of the applicant pool. Attrition, for those enrolled in the nursing major, has dropped. Curricula have become more liberal. All of these changes, related to the educational milieu and its processes, have occurred as we have settled into the mainstream of higher education.

One very positive influence on nursing education, which may have simultaneously promoted and benefited from our independence of hospital dominance, is our system of specialized accreditation. Since the late 1940s, first the National Nursing Accrediting Service (NNAS) and shortly thereafter in 1952 the National League for Nursing have served very effectively as the instrument for peer review of schools of nursing. Through this means, which has become a model to other professions, we have been able to set and enforce quality criteria for nursing education, to shape and bolster our position in the collegiate environment, and to exert additional self-governance. (Unfortunately, we have not been able to achieve a similar goal in hospital nursing services, because we have been virtually without control of the standard-setting function within the processes of the Joint Commission on Accreditation of Hospitals.)

What about the effect of our affiliation with academia on *product?* This is somewhat equivocal. Many nursing service directors complain about the graduates of collegiate nursing programs, and some refuse to employ them without additional seasoning. Increased clinical experience pregraduation and internships postgraduation are repeatedly proposed. Nurses continue to drop out of the field as a result of job dissatisfaction. On the other side of the ledger, significant numbers remain in nursing, perform quite well, report that their education has prepared them adequately, and are bringing new leadership to nursing; employers often say these newcomers to the field are the best ever.

Overall, though, it is impractical to deny possible negative consequences to nursing education's independence from nursing service and the concomitant embracing of the ideals of education. *Two* are uppermost in my mind.

First, serious problems have developed over the lack of articulation, even communication, between the academic and practice branches. One outcome, reality shock in the recent graduate, is best described and documented in Marlene Kramer's study on the subject (14). The concept of accountability, which is popular in our current thinking, somehow does not seem to extend to the relationship between our two vital professional components. Neophyte nurses and a badly served public are caught in the chasm that has opened up. Recent efforts are being made to remedy this defect. Some health science centers are experimenting with organizational patterns for achieving closer collaboration or reintegration between the two enterprises.

Although the preceding concern related to the bifurcation of nursing into education and service is a universal one, I may be worrying alone on the *second,* resulting, I believe, from our having in larger measure substituted the discipline of education for the discipline of nursing. It seems to me that we have displaced the balance between curriculum development and the substance of instruction; that the pedagogical emphasis has eclipsed, rather than served, the critical clinical science foundation. With respect to the former, we have surpassed our masters in the field of education.

It is not unusual to find course syllabi that are voluminous masterpieces, often the result of untold hours of effort by individuals or teaching teams or curriculum committees and sometimes replacing textbooks in the field. Nevertheless, faculty are teaching in areas in which they or others have not done much research and, frequently, in which their clinical expertise is tenuous. Therefore, the instruction relies heavily on opinion and conjecture, generously passed around in the literature, on outside experiences and role models, and on processes—nursing process, change process, communication process, decision process, research process, leadership process, discovery process, and process process.

The use of process as didactic content most likely stems from our ties to education. Assuredly, it is sound—to an extent. But it becomes costly self-deception at the extreme where the process is confused with or substituted for the event, a practice described by linguists as nominalization (6:14). Further, just as process cannot replace event, conceptual frameworks, valuable in giving unity and organization to a curriculum, nevertheless cannot replace the science of the discipline.

Yet, with all they do, faculty admittedly are already over-burdened. Adding scientific inquiry and the maintenance of clinical skills to the existing emphasis on curriculum and instruction is to overtax a bulging schedule. However, it is becoming more and more apparent that universities intend to exact the full academic role—teaching, research, and university and community service—of nurses admitted to regular faculty status. This creates for nurse educators a dilemma that, more than any other, reflects the alien backgrounds and the clashing values of the profession and the "pure" disciplines. Our health service motives, our commitment to our human "laboratories," compel us to make agonizing choices in our university homes, where the ground rules have been set by generations of venerable academicians. We are pulled by two poles, sometimes in conflict, and in combination, imposing inordinate demands on us.

How can we meet both professional and academic mandates? We might do so by recognizing the true compatibilities of the two worlds and by melding the promising features of both, some of which are touched on below.

Clinical, nontenure tracks are reluctantly being developed in some schools to provide the clinical arm of instruction. This movement deserves cautious appraisal, for it may meet one need while worsening others. On the one hand, it provides students with access to clinical experts and role models who, for reasons of preparation, priority, or proclivity, do not engage in research in a major way. On the other hand, it may reduce the pressures and resources for critical development of the knowledge base of the discipline. On the whole though, it perpetuates an unhealthy pluralism in attitude and practice.

Also, it may mute nursing's voice in the governance of the university, since clinical faculty seldom possess full faculty rights.

So efforts must be redoubled to test additional approaches to extending faculty resources; for example, a freer exchange with service counterparts; the use of graduate students as instructional and research assistants; teaching assignments adjusted to the ebb and flow of particular research projects; consolidating courses and classes into larger, less frequent offerings; streamlining teaching methods; clustering research interests; encouraging collaborative projects; reducing committee and counseling responsibilities; increasing independence for students; and others. Both faculty and students may welcome and benefit from such changes, some of which have long been respected in academia but have been foreign or contrary to our traditions and convictions in nursing education. As faculty in nursing, steeped in the nurturance culture of our gender and profession, we sometimes find it difficult to liberate students to explore their own paths to self-actualization and professional competence.

Students, as well as practicing colleagues, often fail to appreciate the importance of the multifaceted role of the professional in universities. Undergraduates, especially, resent the "irrelevant" distractions from teaching of their professors who take time for scientific investigation and writing. Also students are often scornful of perceived clinical inadequacies of faculty and frequently form their attachments to and identification with practitioners in the service setting. To some extent, this attitude may be "caught" from faculty who, on occasion, speak of research expectations like doing time in the French Foreign Legion—alien, isolated, and punitive. The pressures of competing demands have made them appear unaware, for the moment, that, without findings from scientific investigation, they have no indigenous nursing material to teach—or to practice.

The fostering of *collegiality* in students and the problem of juggling the components of the faculty role may both be partially amenable to the same solution—that of developing the concept of the "community of professional scholars." This term is used to designate a partnership in learning, practice, and research that binds and magnifies the dimensions of faculty, students, clinicians, and heightens their sense of accomplishment and self-worth. Herein, *faculty* will find a meshing in the components of their role and will be assisted by the contributions of student and practitioner colleagues in aspects of its fulfillment. Herein, *students* will best understand collegiality and appreciate scientific inquiry, as they are caught up in faculty-practitioner investigations and experience science as a basis for their education and practice. Herein, *clinicians* will continue to be a part of and influenced by a learning environment. And, herein, the pace of the development and dissemination of the *research* base for practice will be accelerated. Thus, ultimacy and collegiality and role fulfillment are simultaneously served.

We should wish most mightily for the day that the twin concepts of "community of scholars" and "lifelong learning" inflame both the university and the professions and that they replace the education-practice segmentation and the start-stop system of basic-advanced-continuing education. The imposition of continuing education requirements for relicensure and the refusal of public universities to subsidize continuing education are bold evidence that these notions have not caught hold.

Selected issues in nursing curricula

The earlier part of this chapter offered general commentary about professions and academia and broad influences in nursing education. These translate into particular issues confronting schools as they make critical administrative and programmatic decisions. I have selected six major themes for discussion here. All relate directly or indirectly to the fundamental concerns about professional education enumerated earlier and establish once again that nursing is, in its own peculiar way, experiencing the developmental pains common to the professions.

To set out on a positive note, accord seems to have been reached on the *purpose of schools of nursing.* They exist (1) to generate knowledge through research and (2) to socialize students to the norms, values, and roles of the profession and provide them with the knowledge and skills essential for developing and performing socially beneficial and self-actualizing roles as nurses. Difficulties and disaccord are more likely to arise over the specific *objectives,* in terms of knowledge, skills, values, traits, and roles and, perhaps to an even greater extent, over the *means* to their attainment. I would like to quickly survey those themes of controversy of which I am most aware and about which I feel most intensely, beginning with that which may be most fundamental and most serious.

A diverse professional body for a diverse clientele. One of the general issues in professional education, identified on page 157, refers to the need for competent professionals to serve diverse clients. The assumption has been made that this requires a similarly diverse student body, reasoning that professionals will better understand and be more committed to the care of persons from socioeconomic, ethnic, and racial backgrounds like their own, as well as more readily gain their acceptance and cooperation.

Nursing's interest in disadvantaged groups, while hardly complete and not without some apathy and resistance, was established early and with greater success than in other health professions. Nursing has had a proud history of going into ghettos to care for the poor and of militantly championing their social welfare. Nursing schools opened their doors to blacks before federal mandate and proceeded to actively recruit minorities. Awards and scholarships have been established nationally and locally to recognize and encourage such efforts. However, according to 1977 statistics, only 2.5 percent of the profession are black (2:28), and there is only slight encouragement in knowing that a mere 4.7 percent of the 1978 graduating class were so identified (19:37). Hispanics have historically been underrepresented in nursing. One conjecture about the decline in minority entrants into nursing is that potential applicants have been attracted to other fields previously unfriendly to women and ethnic minorities.

Too many men continue to shun nursing and may sometimes feel that they are shunned by nursing. Only 2.0 percent of nurses practicing in 1977 were male (2:3). There may be cause for optimism about a gradual increase, in that 6 percent of nursing students admitted to all basic R.N. programs in 1977-1978 were men (19:25).

As the Bakke case, charging "reverse" discrimination against a Caucasian applicant to medical school, was being argued in the courts, it was feared that a judgment might be rendered that would adversely affect affirmative action programs. In the 1978 ruling of the U.S. Supreme Court, quotas were denounced, but special consideration of race in admissions procedures was reaffirmed (11:481). It may still be too early to tell—in fact, we may never know—the impact of this bitter debate and the decision on the aspirant pool, as well as on school policies.

Admission requirements constitute only one of the factors affecting the matriculation of the disadvantaged in nursing programs. Financial assistance, disastrously dwindling, is especially critical to this group. Academic and social support systems are also of major importance. And, referring back to the earlier chapters on the cardinal attributes for professionhood in nursing, we may ask: What is the source of collegiality for such students?

Our responsibility to a diverse body of clients goes beyond achieving a diverse body of professionals. It must extend into curriculum plans and clinical experiences that take cognizance of the particular needs of all segments of society. And research must supply this information.

Nursing's corporate body, as well as individual schools, are challenged to intensify efforts to provide "professionals prepared for practice in a changing world of diverse clients" (page 157).

General education versus professional education. How much of each and in what sequence should liberal and career-specific education be applied? NLN criteria and basic baccalaureate curricula tend to favor a fifty-fifty distribution between the two, with the nursing half on top. The generic master's (M.N.) and doctoral (N.D.) programs in nursing, like educational programs in the other professions such as medicine, dentistry, theology, and law, build the professional component on a four-year general education base. Challenging this position is Spurr's authoritative treatise for the Carnegie

Commission, *Academic Degree Structures: Innovative Approaches,* which asserts that:

> While there is general acceptance that the student trained both in the general liberal arts and in a specific field of concentration or in a specific profession is more desirably educated than either the pure generalist or the pure specialist, it is by no means clear that one phase of education should be separated in time from the other or, if so, which should precede which. To be specific, it is not desirable to confine general liberal arts education to the first two years and subject-matter specialization to the last two years of undergraduate study. In many cases, it is better to allow the student who is preoccupied with a given line of study to follow this line vigorously in his first exposure to the university, as long as his program will be balanced out before he finishes. (22)

There are pious opinion and tradition on both sides of the issue. Where would curriculum research put its weight in the debate? It is especially important that we know because, along with levels of nursing practice, there are emerging two distinct paths in nursing education—generic and incremental. Some students go directly into baccalaureate and higher degree programs; some work their way up the ladder. At the heart of the controversy is the sequencing of the liberal and professional content. What are the effects of various educational patterns on competence and on socialization—the two purposes for nursing education mentioned earlier?

Generalization versus specialization. The range of opinion along the generalization-specialization continuum is manifested both in instructional methodology and program design and in basic and advanced nursing education. This issue underlies such long-standing arguments as to whether schools should teach facts and procedures, by repetition, or principles and concepts, by inquiry and discovery. On another level, this theme is evident in the wide variations among undergraduate curricula, some with one common set of nursing courses for all students; others encouraging early interest-testing or specialization through electives, areas of concentration, or even separate paths such as the episodic and distributive tracks recommended in *An Abstract for Action* by the National Commission for the Study of Nursing and Nursing Education (16). Graduate programs in nursing also reflect uncertainty on this issue of generalization versus specialization and particularly on the matter of relative emphasis on the clinical and functional aspects. Should more attention be paid to the substantive nursing content or to the role development requirements for teaching, administration, and so forth?

In recent years, this has become a larger social issue, with medicine as the major focus of attention. The trend toward overspecialization is said to create demand, fragment care, increase costs, and be motivated by provider aggrandizement rather than service enhancement. We should keep a watchful eye out for the effects of the certification movement in nursing on the future development of the profession with respect to specialization.

New graduate as master technician and manager versus neophyte professional. What are the legitimate performance expectations of the beginning practitioner? As was acknowledged previously, the discrepant views of the school and the employer regarding the competencies and attitudes of nurses emerging fresh from the educational environment is a topic of frequent concern, with serious ramifications. In the debate, the practice branch argues that graduates aren't prepared for the rigors of nursing today. Nursing education rebuts that the system is preparing nurses to create and function within a dynamic, improved health care system.

Many nursing service directors concede that it is unreasonable to expect that practitioners highly skilled for all settings will emerge from the educational system. Yet complaints persist about the new graduates' lack of both *technical* and *leadership* skills—opposite ends of the functional spectrum. "They can't catheterize" and "they can't supervise" are common allegations exemplifying the versatility and breadth characteristic of nursing. As was mentioned earlier, the question of adding an internship to basic programs, to enable the development of these heroic proportions, surfaces periodically. The proposal meets with objections from those who view it as unnecessary or leading to possible exploitation of graduate nurses or as being too close to the "medical model."

Schools and health care agencies, alike, await the outcome of the ANA 1978 resolution to establish competencies for baccalaureate and associate degree graduates (3:9). Such an approach holds promise for reconciling the conflicting "prepare for what is" and the "prepare for what should be" positions generally held by nursing service and nursing education, respectively.

Primary versus tertiary care. This title, an oversimplification, is intended to embrace a broad range of *role and purpose variables* and is related to the preceding controversy about *performance variables.* Such a grab bag contains the entire range of uncertainties about the nature of nursing, as it appeared on page 96 in the discussion of "The Meaning of Our Work." This lack of consensus, as we would expect, is evident in curriculum endeavors. Are schools to prepare students for primary, secondary, or tertiary care? For hospitals, communities, or homes? To promote wellness or to tend the critically ill? To be good thinkers, planners, coordinators, managers, or bedside nurses? To be independent, dependent, or interdependent? Is nursing some or all of these? What is the nuclear role required of each beginning nurse?

These persistent questions stress the need for a clear statement about the nature of nursing, which the ideology (page 61) undertook in a broad way, taking the position that, indeed, we are all of the above. Rather than continuing the debate, we could apply our energies to establishing the fundamental education base and the means to its furtherance after graduation.

The mysteries of socialization. What values do students bring to their nursing programs? What values, norms, roles, and symbols do they learn in nursing schools? What should be the objectives of the socialization process and when and how are these best achieved?

More than fifteen years ago Ingeborg Mauksch analyzed twenty-eight studies of personality factors found in nurses. The findings:

> A high need for succorance
> > submissiveness
> > order, and
> > blame avoidance
> A low need for risk-taking. (17:1296)

It is not known to what extent these characteristics might turn up in surveys today. But to the extent that they exist, they would not make anyone's list of attributes for the well turned out or well–turned on professional. Seeing them enumerated in such fashion does point out the need for special attention to be given to both the selection and the instructional processes in nursing education. But, first, schools are faced with the need to identify those behaviors and values they wish to foster. These, too, should emerge from beliefs about nursing.

As you know from Section Five, I would be most concerned that the overarching attitudes of *social signficance,* *ultimacy* of professional performance, and *collegiality/collectivity* be developed. In their respective chapters, those qualities were defined and brief references to their development were made. But, another book—volumes, in fact—could be devoted to research on the subject and the means of acquiring these and other values. Later in our venture key elements in an effective socialization relationship will be considered.

The issues outlined here must not be treated just as minor difficulties or friendly family squabbles. They represent serious professional weaknesses with serious consequences. We see the disastrous results in (1) confusion and disillusionment for the individual *nurse;* (2) attrition from the field and lack of control for the nursing *profession;* and (3) less-than-our-best-effort for the *public.*

A WORD (OR TWO) IN CLOSING

In this chapter a bit of optical juggling has been attempted. Nursing education has been examined through binocular lenses, shifting between a general outlook on professional education, derived from Section Two literature, at one eye, and the nursing ideology, expounded in Section Three, at the other.

Looking at nursing through the professional education looking glass, we found that, more often than not, the images merged. That is, on the whole, issues in nursing reflect the basic issues in professional education, although nursing has lagged and demonstrated its own eccentricities in its course into and through academia. Questions about values, roles, methods, admissions, performance standards, beginning practice competencies, and liberalization versus specialization, often rising out of the academic-practice dichotomy, are as cogent and pressing in nursing as in other applied fields, if not more so. This wide-angle lens has registered the if, how, and why nursing is like or unlike other professions, on the whole. Ideals or goals have not entered this picture. It has descriptively dealt with the "what is," not prescriptively with the "what should be." This second mission has been left to the ideological eye.

The ideological eye inspected the blurred uncertainties about nursing education and brought them into focus with its conviction about the nature and purpose of our work. This perspective has applied more to the broad ends of education—that is, preparation for the clinical science, humanism, and technology of nursing and the acquisition of the attitudes requisite for its fulfillment—and less to the specific means toward their accomplishment. This gives us pause to note that the ideological emphasis on essence and ends is appropriate in that it grants many degrees of freedom in the pursuit of the goals of nursing education, yet it points out just as aptly that the outcome is the real proof of the educational process.

The concluding discussion of selected issues did not explicitly refer to the ideology for guidance. However, we can see that the beliefs stand ready to chart a particular course as challenges are posed. For example, with respect to the generalization-specialization questions, how can the wide-ranging goals of "humanism" and the management of nursing's "organizational, legal, economic, and political" context best be served through education? And, on the primary versus tertiary debate, how can nursing's "concern for all persons, all human health states," and in all settings best be served through education?

If this act of optical legerdemain has succeeded at all in its ambition, we should possess both a close and contextual view of nursing education today, as well as some prospects for a happier future. If it has not succeeded in the attempt, we can turn the page and ponder how a misstep may have occurred.

19

REFLECTIONS ON
A MISCONCEPTION

Originally, this section on *The Foundations of Nursing Practice* was designed to comprise two chapters entitled "Nursing Education" and "Nursing Research." I wrote and rewrote and reorganized and revised and . . . . No amount of fussing or fretting could make it work.

In the first place, the passages on EDUCATION that you have just read were essentially preaching or rehashing our troubled past. When I realized what had happened, I modified the title to admit this limitation and rearranged some of the material, unquestionably an action more cosmetic than corrective in effect. But I chose to do this rather than eliminate the chapter because it assists us in ventilating some feeling that we all have about education—our own and that of the currently muddled system—and it puts some aspects in general and historical perspective.

Then I encountered a second problem. When time came to write about RESEARCH, preaching turned to probing. Or, to switch metaphors, a monsoon on one subject was followed by a drought on another. (A book for all seasons!) Admittedly, scientific endeavor is the area in which my own background is most sadly lacking. I have no mental reservoir bursting with knowledge, experience, and emotion; no pencilled hand eager to spill out the contents, as was true with education. On the contrary, this "probing" on research began with reading and reading and reading on the subject: a searching, unsettled mind; still fingers. I agonized: What could a relative novice add to the writings on nursing research? A six-page bibliography? A summary? An accounting of issues and problems? A synthesis? A particular insight? A new angle? An original paradigm or theory? A treatise on values?

After I reminded myself that the intent of the book is socialization, not erudition, I realized that I could take advantage of my shortcoming, rather than strain it. I could capitalize on the likelihood that my personal development in research approximates the professional mean and thus enables me to probe the scientific aspect of the nursing universe through my own sentiments and hunches in a representative fashion.

I inclined first toward a bit of rightful, but not very productive, self-ridicule and breast-beating: Could it be believed that we have descended from "the passionate statistician" Florence Nightingale, who used facts and figures to understand and explain health phenomena, to recommend treatments, to persuade government officials?

And then the puzzlement: From these roots, how did we grow to believe that instinct, ritual, feeling, and obedience to others could combine to make a *total, trustworthy* response to the complex human health condition? How have we come to accept not knowing, to the extent that knowing is possible, the probabilities that one of our "merciful" acts will benefit the patient more than another, or even that it will do him no harm?

This fruitless rummaging for explanations provoked an equally fitful reaching out for remedies: What can be said to move us to fully integrate into our self-concepts the intellectual curiosity of the scientist coupled with the practical responsibility of the professional? How can the near-blind selection of treatment modalities be made intolerable to us? What will bring us to the proper realization that practice without verified knowledge must soon be considered unethical? When will we truly understand that we have no freedom to act on our own expert authority until we have developed the science to warrant independent action? How can we be convinced that scientific investigation is not the last thing to be done but the first thing to be done? Where is the Wizard who will graft the mind of the researcher to the heart and hands of the nurse? What? How? When? Where? All searching for solutions.

To regain my bearings, I proceeded to consider where the philosophical and attitudinal base we have been building throughout the book would lead. The *beliefs* on the nature and purpose of nursing declare ends to be achieved and indicate general directions to be pursued (page 61). Research to improve the quality of life through nursing care is a major means—the stepping stone—to the achievement of those goals. Our sense of *social significance* would tell us this is so. Our sense of *ultimacy* of professional performance would impel us to utilize this critical means and would point out where the needs are greatest. Our sense of *collegiality* would urge us to construct our own scientific contributions with, for, and on the work of our colleagues in this shared pursuit.

When I reached this point, I could image the clamor of voices protesting that beliefs and attitudes aren't the problem. Time, resources, expertise, policies, incentives are the problem! I say these things myself. I hear others repeat them. I read them in the literature. Such extrinsic factors are undeniably *influences* and *obstacles*. But my conviction is that the *problem* is indeed the intrinsic underlying one of individual characteristics and attitudes, compounded by professional norms, values, and roles—a combination resulting from selection into the field and the socialization thereafter. In a possible cause-and-effect debate on this issue, I am persuaded, perhaps from my own example, that we can and will tear down the external barriers to scientific investigation when we are sufficiently motivated to do so and when we understand the nature of the fundamental problems. Yet the effect of the institutional characteristics on research attitudes and productivity, whether primary or secondary in importance, must not be discounted.

Socialization and motivation—personal, intrinsic factors—popping up in a fundamental discussion of research? There I was back on the doorstep of the nursing school. But recognizing also that the influences of the practice environment need, too, to be shaped and "socialized" in reciprocal fashion. Eureka! The original error in the concept of the two chapters, proposing to treat education and research in sequential fashion and independent of the institutional context in which they exist, was unmistakable. The realization that I was succumbing to and perpetuating a fundamental source of our professional weakness was startling.

But the proper direction was clear. The concept of a new endowment for nursing, based on an understanding of the inextricable relationships among our *developmental and functional tasks* and their *surroundings*, flew into my mind and would not be dislodged. The book—suddenly nearing completion—first received its name. And this chapter, only now recognized as the culmination of this uncharted journey, was retitled "Articulated Professional, Academic, Socialization, and Governance Models for a New Endowment" and was committed to a revised trajectory, one that treats these cornerstones of nursing practice in their true interdependent relationship. One that looks, not back in anger and alarm but forward in hope and determination, to the birth—or more accurately, the birthing—of a new generation. For those of us already in the field, becoming part of this new generation requires dramatic changes. For those yet to be ushered in, some major initiatives must be launched.

As this section proceeds, it will become apparent that attention is focused on the advanced levels of nursing education and practice. This stems from the belief that, as the profession progresses to its greatest performance, maximum effort must be concentrated on this growing edge. As the anguish of the segment on nursing education's troubled past attested, I am painfully aware that programs preparing for beginning technical and professional practice must continue to search for their *métier* and actualize in relation to one another. That process is not to be ignored but will be affected by the speed, direction, and extent to which nursing spirals to higher levels of capacity and achievement, the struggle in which we have long been engaged and in which we are honor bound by our social contract to persist. The struggle that has caused us to add new knowledge, skill, role, and value planes to nursing, as emerging health needs and means have been identified and developed, and the profession accordingly continues to be reshaped.

20

ARTICULATED PROFESSIONAL, ACADEMIC, SOCIALIZATION, AND GOVERNANCE MODELS FOR A NEW ENDOWMENT

THE SIGNIFICANCE OF THE NEW ENDOWMENT

What is the new endowment? The word "endowment" was chosen here for its abundant meaning. It was chosen to express the investment of fresh perspective, natural capacity, and power in ourselves—in nursing. It was chosen to connote the bestowal of a dower, or permanent provision of support, on our professional progeny. Specifically, within the intent of this writing, the phrase *new endowment* refers to the values, resources, modes and means, and relationships that together will enlarge our present capacities, will further evolve the intrinsic makeup or "gene pool" of our descendants, and will bring added dimensions to our societal contributions, which thus enrich our public legacy.

This act of re-creation involves an appreciation that our future depends on overcoming a principal deficit—that is, our failure to develop in a coordinated, reciprocal manner our tasks, both developmental and operational, and their environment to achieve a "fit" or articulation among them. By *developmental tasks*, I am referring to education, socialization, and research; by *operational tasks*, I am referring to nursing practice, broadly defined. By *environment*, I am referring to the sociopolitical and organizational context within which both sets of tasks occur.

This act of re-creation also involves the restoration of discarded principal as well as the reinvestment of healthy, active principal. For example, we must begin by removing from the recesses of discredited history and exposing to the light of objective reappraisal such words and concepts as *apprenticeship, training, dependency,* and *medical model.* All were rejected at one time for their undesirable features, their excesses, and their negative effect on nursing's development; they have continued to be the pariahs of our professional lexicon. Yet each contains some positive aspects that we should be open to reinstate within our assets. Elements having to do with informal, on-site, sometimes repetitive, often inconvenient, ill-defined, and untidy action-problem-content-service oriented learning. Elements having to do with close, personal, hierarchy-of-expertise, mentor-mentee, patron-protege relationships with competent, experienced, established, recognized clinicians, teachers, researchers, and administrators—professionals in nursing and other fields who may or may not be faculty members governed by the university and by narrow educational standards and objectives.

MODELS FOR THE NEW ENDOWMENT

In a very selective fashion, I am proposing models that will contribute to the new endowment. Models that to some extent recapture and exemplify these lost elements just mentioned, interspersed with the fundamental attitudes of social significance, ultimacy, and collegiality, and that reflect the clinical science, technology, and humanism of nursing's essential nature. For convenience of presentation only, I have categorized these as *professional and academic, socialization,* and *governance* models, but to think of them as discrete entities would be to defeat our mutuality and ecological thesis. Also, as you will see, the term "model" is used here in a variety of ways and in a more popular than literal or technical sense.

Within this arbitrary typology, *professional and academic* models are concerned broadly with professional role constructions and with the associated academic degrees, programs, structures, and resources of university nursing schools. *Socialization* models focus on the processes of acquiring the values and expectations of the multifaceted nursing role, an obligation shared by both the academic and practice branches of the profession. *Governance* models deal with the means and modes of professional-institutional interaction and accommodation for standard setting and policymaking in the practice setting—a problem emphasized in the review of the literature. I prefer the term "governance" to autonomy and independence because, in its neutrality, it does not prejudge the mode of interaction and is open to all possible means of establishing and simultaneously achieving institutional and professional objectives.

At first glance governance may seem an unlikely component of this trilogy; it is in fact not only a legitimate but a necessary member, one of both cause and effect in its relationship to the others. For not only must governance be shaped by the new socialization, but it is the vehicle within which this socialization is maximally expressed in nursing practice. Stated another way, with renewed motivation and potential, we *will* develop the mechanisms that enable us to engage the fullness of our capacities in our impact on health care. In a broader sense, one might consider governance models to be practice or clinical models. However, again I prefer the concept of governance, to fix on the context of the expertise, rather than the expertise itself—not to value expertise less, but to recognize that it requires *institutionalized advocacy* to flourish.

Heretofore nursing has devoted considerably more attention to the development of academic programs and professional roles than to the ecology required for their full effect. Stark illustrations of this two-legged stool approach are the clinical specialist and nursing practitioner initiatives, which have suffered significantly from the failure to define, assert, and achieve the clear organizational policies to implement these ideals. Our failures to fully develop this governance aspect in total congruence with educational programs and professional roles may well be our most serious mistake.

Professional and academic models

I drew heavily on the term "advanced clinical scientist" in the chapter on nursing education. This concept provokes questions about whether, in a practical or ideal sense, this is an integrated role embodied in one individual, or complementary roles fulfilled by collaborators. And, too, what about the added dimension of the teaching role?

The hyphen and the slash are the symbols of these conceptualizations—the hyphen combining, the slash separating and relating. Should we aim to be clinician-scientists or clinicians/scientists; clinician-scientist-educators or clinicians/scientists/educators? Emerging from the answers to these questions are the academic models that best prepare for these roles—models that ultimately lead to the identification and investigation of problems and phenomena of nursing concern, to the application of this verified knowledge in practice and its transmission in education. Let us hold these questions in abeyance for the moment and quickly survey nursing's current scene in graduate education.

The dominant pattern in master's degree education in nursing is preparation in an area of clinical specialization. Combined with, and in some instances superseding, this emphasis, there may be functional or role development components in administration, teaching, and others. Research courses are prevalent and a thesis or research project may be required. However, most commonly a research "consumer" or "collaborator," rather than independent investigator, is the avowed intent of the research training* in the curriculum at this level.

While master's education may have settled in, controversy and confusion seem to have risen to the doctoral level. The major issues are: (1) Should the nurse be prepared in nursing or in a basic science, or—an option with mercurial support—in an applied field such as education or administration? (2) What are the comparative purposes, programs, and advantages of "professional doctorates" and "research doctorates" in nursing? As was acknowledged earlier, the federally funded Nurse Scientist program welcomed many nurses into the social and natural sciences during the past two decades. This subsequently gave impetus to the accelerated growth of our own doctoral programs in the 1970s, relying heavily on nurse faculty doctorally prepared in related fields teaming with master's-educated nurse clinicians to supervise doctoral research, a

---

*Whew! It feels so good to be able to use this quite respectable member of the English vocabulary again.

bootstrap operation that may persist for some time. This movement has advanced to the point where postdoctoral fellows have begun to appear in larger numbers.

Professional or research doctorates? The past ten years have produced the original N.D. program, leading to a first professional degree, and increased the D.N.Sc.* programs to seven and the Ph.D. to fourteen (18). It is argued, on the one hand, that professional programs should prepare expert practitioners and users of research (9). Others disagree and describe the D.N.Sc. as the degree for clinical researchers. Still another point of view is that no true professional doctoral program producing clinicians *par excellence* has as yet been developed (12), but that such programs are going the way of the Ph.D., in content if not in name. If so, this may be true either because the Ph.D. is the politically thwarted preference of the schools offering the clinical doctorate or because the Ph.D. programs have not yet yielded the nursing science base necessary for more sophisticated practice. As far as academic preparation for university teaching is concerned, opinion ranges among advocacy of education, the basic sciences, the nursing Ph.D., and the D.N.Sc., depending on whether the emphasis is to be put on pedagogy, basic research, clinical research, or practice expertise.

A gross oversimplification of the issues relating to graduate education in and for nursing! But adequate as a basis for recalling the questions raised earlier about integrated versus parallel roles and for developing answers and academic models from those answers.

Professional roles. To remind ourselves, the question about

---

*A variety of symbols represent the doctorate in nursing science or the science of nursing.

roles was: clinician-scientist-educator or clinician/scientist/educator? The idealist in me argues for the complete clinical scholar, as the most efficacious model for accomplishing our goals. The pragmatist in me recognizes that persons of such heroic proportions are rare, despite the fact that university promotion policies often demand the hero. This leads me to conclude that alternative professional models and alternative academic pathways are supportable, at least until we are clearly convinced that one is far superior to the other. However, in deciding among these models, a major consideration must be to accelerate the development of the clinical science base, which underlies all hope of professional progress.

The professional models I speak of here are those individuals or combinations of persons fulfilling the professional roles of expert scientist, teacher, or practitioner for the generation, transmission, and application of knowledge in the field. The individual who engages in these roles in an *integrated* or *unitary* fashion would be a doctorally prepared nurse who is directly or indirectly responsible for a client case load and is engaged in research and teaching on a regular basis. A variation of this multifaceted professional model would be the individual who carries out these functions alternately rather than concurrently—for example, shifting emphases throughout the academic year. It is not intended to convey that this rounded individual works in isolation, only that she is capable and personally involved in all domains. Another set of professional models would reflect a *parallel* or *complementary* approach, whereby researchers collaborate with clinicians to identify and study problems and disseminate their findings; whereby practitioners team with academicians to serve as clinical preceptors, and so forth.

Academic models. The academic models associated with

these professional models would be, in the first instance of the *integrated clinical scientist,* the D.N.Sc., as most commonly defined as the clinical research degree, or the combination of the M.S. or M.N. specialist degrees or the N.D. with the Ph.D. in nursing or basic sciences. In the second instance of *teaming or complementarity,* the Ph.D. in nursing or a related science (or the D.N.Sc., if soundly research-based) would prepare the research scholar partners; and the M.S., M.N., or N.D. would prepare the clinician and clinical teacher partners. (One must recognize in all of this idealizing that the distinctions between the D.N.Sc. and Ph.D. in nursing are currently blurred in actuality, if not in theory. With few exceptions, research to develop knowledge underlying nursing practice is the objective of programs conferring both degrees.)

Since the syntax is especially garbled in this instance, this may be the place for some diagrammatic relief:

ASSOCIATED PROFESSIONAL AND
ACADEMIC MODELS FOR ROUNDING OUT
THE ADVANCED PROFESSIONAL ROLE TODAY

Comprehensive approaches	Professional models	Academic models
Alternative 1 (integrated)	Clinician-scientist-teacher	D.N.Sc. or combination of M.S., M.N., N.D. with the Ph.D. in nursing or related science
Alternative 2 (parallel)	Researchers and teachers	D.N.Sc. or Ph.D. in nursing or related science
	Clinicians and clinical teachers	M.S., M.N., or N.D.

Schools, in making critical decisions about which programs to offer, and nurses, in deciding which to select, are both weighing need, demand, interest, and resource factors in these institutional and personal deliberations. From the perspective of the profession and the services it is to perform, I believe *we must go back to the knowledge base as the fundamental consideration and thus promote initially those programs and enrollments that have the greatest potential for leading to its development,* whether these be the Ph.D. either in nursing or in the basic sciences with close ties to nursing, or the research-based D.N.Sc. programs. As this body of clinical science grows, it should appear in associate degree, baccalaureate, and graduate curricula in nursing in accordance with the competencies required of those graduates. This swelling body of knowledge should push up the educational level for entry into professional practice and should fill out the true professional doctorates, rather than the reverse— namely, inflating the educational standard and goal beyond the scientific content to warrant and sustain them.

It is intriguing to consider that the ultimate outcome of such a content-driven approach to practice roles and academic program development—and, incidentally, to licensing and certification—could be an academic schema incorporating the associate degree (or even the baccalaureate in time) for the "technical" or "nurse associate" level; the N.D. for professional practice; the N.D.-Ph.D. combination, similar to the medical scientist model, for the clinical researcher; and the M.S. and D.N.Sc. becoming the steps for the upwardly mobile nurse from the current cohort of those prepared at the baccalaureate level. I expect we will also begin to see merging of the professional master's and doctoral programs, as has occurred in other disciplines in which the doctorate has become the terminal degree, and concomitantly the stress on research will be at the doctoral level. This futuristic model could be depicted in the following way:

FUTURISTIC CONTENT-DRIVEN ACADEMIC MODELS INCLUDING GENERIC AND TRANSITIONAL INCREMENTAL ROUTES PREPARING FOR PROFESSIONAL PRACTICE AND THE CLINICAL SCIENTIST/ACADEMICIAN ROLES

Educational routes	Professional practitioner	Clinical scientist-academician
Generic route B.S. in liberal arts ⟶	N.D.* or M.N.*	
Transitional incremental route B.S.N.* ⟶ M.S.N. ⟶ or B.S.N.* ⟶	D.N.Sc. or M.S.N.-D.N.Sc. (merged)	Ph.D.

*First professional degrees.

Specialization, which will be of increasing importance with an expanding base of knowledge and technology, could occur within the upper levels of the incremental route, as is now the case, or during the M.N. or N.D. first professional degree programs, or in postgraduate master's specialty programs or residencies. Schools might offer the N.D. (or M.N.) or the N.D.-Ph.D. combination; the M.S. and D.N.Sc. or the D.N.Sc.-Ph.D. combination. Nursing science and nursing practice could be well served in these models.

Innovations in the design of schools should match innovation in the design of programs. For example, medicine has long recognized its reliance on basic sciences. To bring the full attention of these scientists to medicine, they have enfolded them within their institutional structures by creating entire departments of the basic disciplines within medical schools. Physicians hold joint appointments within such departments; medical students study therein, sometimes simultaneously earning the Ph.D.; medical problems receive the full fury of their research efforts; medical science flourishes. Nursing has attempted this courtship of the scientists in more random, less intensive ways, sometimes by contracting with them, sometimes by attracting isolated researchers, often deprived of adequate laboratories and the stimulation of their colleagues. If we are prepared to think of copying successful features from the medical model, this is an interesting one to contemplate—one we could have best taken advantage of during the years of rapid expansion and burgeoning resources for the nursing education enterprise. We should be prepared to exploit the idea if and when another wave of financial largesse occurs.

As a second structural consideration, we might concentrate for a moment on those organizational forms that encourage collaborative research in our field. For the sake of nursing science as well as the survival of the overburdened nurse academician, we need to work together clustering, replicating, and augmenting studies and maximizing resources. Nursing departments established around substantive areas of nursing knowledge and practice, rather than around units for administering curricula (for example, undergraduate and graduate faculty, or integrated course or level teams), is one such facilitative mechanism. Also, our early and unevenly effective propensity for setting up *general research* departments or offices to support and promote the overall research efforts of university nursing schools should soon evolve into *research-specific* institutes or centers similar to those of our colleagues in more mature disciplines. Such research priorities as psychological stress, pain management, quality of life for the aged, and others identified by the WICHE Delphi survey (25) and identified in federal priorities should be good targets for intense, aggregated efforts. Overall, vehicles contributing to research *density* and *depth* rather than *diversification* should be encouraged while our science is in its infancy and our scientists are in precious supply.

The matter of our researchers being tied into the practice setting has already been discussed in the chapter on nursing education. Structural and policy considerations for getting scientists into the field and clinicians into the laboratories are pertinent here as well. Suffice it to say, "joint" has tended to express the key mechanisms used—joint appointments, joint programs, joint projects, and joint publications.

This moves us to think about models of socialization that engender shared values, loyalties, and role expectations; mutuality of purpose; and constructive relationships among all of the nursing community. Nursing education and nursing practice colleagues join in this responsibility.

And the new endowment would begin to unfold, with coordinated, coherent, relevant professional and academic models.

Socialization models

In simplest terms, socialization is the process of becoming indoctrinated into the whys and wherefores of the group—in this case, the nursing profession. Learning what the job is, discovering what behaviors are expected and respected, developing relationships and loyalties, finding out how to draw on the group resources.

In a mystical sense, socialization is inhaling, being transformed by, and entering the heady professional ethos that fills and surrounds us. As socializers, we create the atmosphere to be breathed; we assist the socializees through the induction; and we join them in the rich mix of values, roles, and behaviors needed to sustain our work at its highest level of performance. Thus for purposes of clarification and discrimination in the particular typology of this chapter, we could identify that the basic content or substance of the professional models was expertise and roles; that of the academic models, degrees and administrative structures; *the "stuff" of socialization models, whether individuals or programs, is interaction modes throughout the professional sphere.* Herein we can deal with only the most obvious aspects of this interaction. It will not be possible within the length and framework of this discussion to examine those subtle nuances that suffuse the ethos of professional relationship and are perhaps the most active ingredients in the interaction. Although nearly indefinable, they are captured and imprinted on the professional soul through the inner eye.

Objectives and participants. Section Five proposed the major attitudes to be engendered by the socialization process and, while they may not stand alone, these are the objectives I would adopt as the basis for an ambitious program of socialization. The fundamental socialization question then emerges: What relationships and modes of interaction promote these goals? What modes promote the development of the sense of *social significance*, that certainty about the nature and importance of our work, that sense of mission and social sanction? What modes promote *ultimacy of professional performance*, that commitment to doing our utmost in our work? What modes promote *collegiality and collectivity*, that conviction that responsibility and authority are shared and that the wholeness of the profession must be preserved?

And who are the participants in this dramatic transformation into professionhood? Since, as Section Five also mentioned, our professional identity is both inwardly and outwardly validated, the entire universe in its historical dimensions could be declared as party to the socialization process. But, for this brief passage, let us concentrate on the central characters and the immediate situation: students and their peers, faculty, clinical and other professional contacts; schools, health care settings, and nursing organizations.

Elements in the interaction. Perhaps I should stop to explain that my views on socialization are not based on rigorous studies or theories of behavior but on experience, observation, and reflection. They are offered in the spirit of this entire volume—that of inviting you to challenge and improve on them.

It seems to me that for us in our role as socializers—and this includes all of us, junior and senior members of the professional community alike—to have a substantial, constructive, and lasting impact on the professional values, conduct, and self-concept of another, there are several important elements in that relationship. The first and critical underlying component is a psychological state; the others, although attitudinal to some degree, are largely action components emanating from that motivation. These action components are not all present in all relationships and in all interactions; in fact, they may to some extent occur in a developmental sequence as presented. Also, it should be stressed that these elements must deliberately be acknowledged and internalized very personally by the socializer and thus are written here in a form to make this emphasis and to allow space for personal reflection.

We started from page one of this dialogue with the thesis *that the central figure in the mirror of nursing is our own.* Now let us add and turn toward a second figure that we have the opportunity and the obligation to infuse with our shared culture.

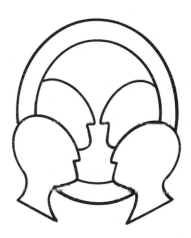

To have an appreciable influence on another member of our professional community, the following elements should enter into our relationship:

Identification

I would identify with her, whether I know her or not. I would feel a close emotional association, a kinship, a colleagueship by virtue of our mutual cause. I would be convinced, and in turn convince her, that we are significant to each other, and that our successes and failures, our pasts and futures, are linked to each other.

Exemplification

I would exemplify those traits, values, processes, and roles that I perceive as deserving to be developed and transmitted in our professional culture. A strong sense of social significance, ultimacy of performance, and collegiality and collectivity would be principal among these attributes.

Instruction

I would teach her, in person and through our professional literature, where and when she needs and wants to be better informed and where I have special knowledge, or experience, or conviction. In turn, I would demonstrate my eagerness to learn from her.

Exemplification would give support and credence to instruction.

Appraisal

I would evaluate her according to my understanding of the standards of professional performance and my perception of her capacities for professional achievement and would constructively inform her of this assessment, reinforcing positive and progressive behavior. I would encourage her self-appraisal. In turn, I would be open to her appraisal of myself.

Sanction

I would ratify her professional conduct, through such academic and professional mechanisms as grades, peer review, credentials, memberships, and privileges.

Collaboration

I would work with her in a collegial manner in learning, practice, research, or other professional endeavors, through joint activity, as well as recognition of and support for her individual accomplishments.

Sponsorship

I would present and certify her to the professional community and to client populations through my practice and contacts, through joint publications, and so forth.

Acculturation

I would acquaint her with the formal and informal mechanisms and the tacit and explicit values of the work environment and assist her to an adjustment that preserves our mutual professional values.

Significance of the elements

Identification,
exemplification,
instruction,
appraisal,
sanction,
collaboration,
sponsorship,
and acculturation

As I look back over these skeletal statements about the key components in the socialization relationship, my eye picks up new angles, new shadings, and new depths in random fashion. These represent only a fraction of those that occur to you, I would hope.

☐ While this discussion consciously focuses on interaction and, more specifically, professional interaction, it must not suggest that socialization occurs solely through this relationship. It is, however, a dominant force that can be deliberately planned and executed and must not be taken lightly.

☐ We all treat professional socialization as a function of time and of repeated exposure or reinforcing circumstance. My spontaneous use of the expression "dramatic transformation" suggests another subject for research—that is, the possible occurrence and nature of socialization as a result of a singular, critical event—sort of along the line of a religious conversion. An anecdotal approach might be used: Have you ever experienced an event that you would characterize as having the predominant, sustaining influence on your acquisition of the professional values and behaviors you possess?

☐ These components can be moved up and down and in and out in level, scale, and scope. For example:

• They apply equally to *individuals* seeking their own ways to carry out their professional responsibility for socialization, or to *programs* set up to achieve the desired ends of socialization within educational or service institutions or professional associations. The term "models," as used here, relates to both.

- They can be viewed as contributing to the development of a "total" nursing role, as discussed in the immediate past segment on professional models, or they can be viewed as useful in fostering the development of particular aspects of that role—for example, scholarship, clinical practice, political acumen, or whatever.

- Expanding beyond the inner sphere of the nursing universe and the conceptualization of these components as the core of the socialization process that shapes the individual member of the profession, it is intriguing to contemplate that, ideally, these components pervade the professional sphere as well. In other words, in referring back to the qualities leading to professionhood, these interactive elements could become the means to collectivity or the sense of community, as well as collegiality, the dyadic relationship.

☐ Have the elements, as described, placed too much emphasis on the activity of the socializer and insufficiently stressed the active participation of the socializee and the reciprocal relationship between the two parties? Identification, for example, is clearly a two-way street. In fact, it may be novel that I have focused on the socializer, whereas usually it is the other way around. Also, has this approach neglected to point out that fortunate individuals may be simultaneously socializer and socializee?

☐ In analyzing the education-service partnership in socialization, is it reasonable to assume that the practice setting has a primary responsibility in socializing to the patient-focused role and the school to the role of nursing in society in a more general way?

☐ I have debated whether to add *encouragement* to the list of active elements in the interaction. Ultimately I decided not to do so with the rationale that while this factor, made up of aspects of reinforcement, stimulation, and inspiration, is an essential ingredient, it is more diffuse than discrete and more in the nature of nuance than definable and describable activity.

□ The effect of numbers must not be ignored. Instruction, appraisal, and sanction may be accomplished with large groups; identification, exemplification, and collaboration may require a smaller circle to be effective. But in any case, the critical aspect is that the process is interpersonal rather than impersonal.

□ In diverse ways these elements may be seen as building blocks within various supportive modes such as *mentoring,* a vertical relationship, and *networking,* a horizontal relationship that seems to follow when one has begun to earn his stripes through the former. I have singled out only these two examples because they have been popularized by the women's movement and are gaining attention in nursing. However, a variety of modes exist and are possible. And rightly so. Breaking new ground might be impeded if mentoring were the only route to socialization. Also an expanding field would otherwise be limited by a shortage of mentors.

□ With respect to specific elements, I found myself jotting down these notes:

• There may be an interesting interplay or tension between *identification* and *appraisal.* Identification may promote the more subjective, close, personal perspective of "shared cause," while appraisal takes on the more detached, objective, distanced, impersonal approach recommended for unbiased evaluation. Focusing exclusively on the latter and purely cognitive skills, as we have often been trained to do, disregards a key aspect of socialization.

• What is the effect of symbols on *identification?* Do caps, pins, uniforms, and ceremonies, for example, influence this process?

• In nursing we have tended to underplay the importance of publications and other forms of scholarly communication in informing (*instructing*) our colleagues. We must increasingly accept, as a professional responsibility, the use of this means, which greatly enlarges our individual scope of influence.

- *Collaboration,* like identification, demands self-extension in a major way. It implies ability and willingness on the part of the socializer to recognize, trust, and invest personal effort and credibility in the capacities of the socializee.

And finally

□ To the extent that these eight elements are soundly and solidly incorporated into socialization processes and programs, the goals of socialization are achievable.

And thus the new endowment would grow through the deliberate, systematic investment by *individuals* and education, practice, and professional *environments* in the process of socializing members to the nursing community.

Governance models

Governance is dictionary defined as "exercise of authority; control; a method or system of government or management" (24). The importance of governance within nursing practice settings derives from every aspect of the ideology, but most directly from the belief:

> ... that nursing's maximum contribution ... is dependent on ... the organizational, legal, economic, social, and political arrangements that enable the full and proper expression of nursing values and expertise.

And belief

> in myself and my nursing colleagues ... in our right to be fulfilled, to be recognized, and to be rewarded as highly valued members of society.

The literature on professions is filled with references to the problems created when professions are practiced within bureaucratic organizations. Rather than repeat those discussions, I would refer you to the brief passage on "Professional Roles and Organizational Necessities" in *The Professions in America.* Therein you will find that Barber cogently identifies the crux of the problem and goes on to give hope for its solution in these statements:

> Whereas professions find the pattern of "colleague control" most suitable, the required pattern of authority for formal organizations is "superordinate control." The former consists of control by peers, the latter of control by superiors. As a result of these different types of required authority, it is inevitable that there be a certain amount of strain when professional roles confront organizational necessities. ...
>
> Inevitable strain exists ... but this does not mean inevitable conflict. For where such inevitable strain is created by dif-

ferent social patterns, a variety of accommodative mechanisms can often be created to reduce the strain or to forestall conflict resulting from the strain that remains. (7:25)

He proceeds to categorize accommodative mechanisms as those establishing differentiated *role* structures, differentiated *authority* structures, and differentiated *reward* structures (7:26).

While operating within bureaucracies is a problem for all professions, it is one that has reached crisis proportions in nursing, largely evidenced in shortages of qualified, permanent, full-time, career-committed staff. Out of frustration, many nurses have capitulated to the values and priorities of the health care settings in which they are employed; others have become "utilizers" of the system (page 103); others have circumvented it by coming in the side door through supplemental nursing registries; others have abandoned acute care institutions for community and educational agencies; others have left nursing for sales or ceramics. Most important, many are attempting to reform the system in varying ways and with varying success. A number of organizational forms have been designed and tested to gain increased control over nursing practice and reward, for example, collective bargaining, primary nursing, clinical ladders, nursing staff bylaws, nursing cooperatives, and contracted services provided by nursing corporations.

As to the specific nature of the complaints, both opinion and research on nursing dissatisfaction abound. For expediency and recency, I would defer to the 1980 report of an investigation of the nursing shortage in Texas. In that study it was determined that nurses "choose to remain outside the work force . . . mainly because of the conditions of work to which [they] are subjected" (23:2). The respondents indicated that the following professional prerogatives were abridged as a result of hospital policies and attitudes:

- Autonomy of practice and respect for the judgment of the professional.
- Determination of standards of quality of care and determination of staffing needs and work schedules to achieve the standards.
- Educational programs and support (financial and time) for updating knowledge and skills.
- Participation with full vote in establishing policy related to patient care, personnel benefits, and working conditions.
- Work responsibilities that are nurse related, with elimination of requirements for nurses to perform tasks that are responsibilities of other services.
- Opportunity for professionals to share expertise with other professionals in other agencies, on hospital time.
- Recognition and personnel benefits comparable to those accorded other health care professionals. (23:7)

Therein we are roundly notified that newly formed organizational models would do well to pay careful attention to these unsatisfied claims to professional rights.

Claims and claimants. *Rights*, however, are just one of a number of factors that systems of institutional-professional governance must take into account. And *nurses* are only one group with legitimate claims to be considered within health care systems.

Along with *rights*, at least three additional factors must be reckoned with:

Rights
Goals (or needs or values, however you wish to view them)
Expertise (the combination of knowledge and skill)
Responsibilities

215

Along with *nurses*, at least five additional claimants have a stake in the action:

Nurses
Patients
The nursing profession
Other professions
The institution
The public

With a slight twist of the kaleidoscope, a matrix falls into place, which in its simplest form would appear as below:

Claimants	Claims			
	Rights	Goals	Expertise	Responsibilities
Nurses	X			
Patients				
Nursing profession	X			
Other professions				
Institutions				
Public				

The grid serves to put into perspective that those seven rights claimed by nurses in the Texas study relate to two cells alone in this vast matrix.

Within this complex it can be seen that one claimant's rights are another claimant's responsibilities. For example, speaking in only the broadest terms: (1) the nurse's *right* to *job satisfaction* is the *responsibility* of the *institution* and the *profession;* and (2) the patient's *right* to competent *nursing care* is the *direct responsibility* of the *nurse* and the *indirect responsibility* of the *profession,* the *institution,* and the *public.* Also, as we are well aware, there is a potential for conflict;

for example, when one claimant asserts that his *expertise* supersedes the goals or rights of another, the concept of a hierarchy of claims is introduced. As another example, there is tension between the public's *goal* of economy and the providers' *responsibility* for quality and the client's *goal* of comprehensive care.

Even the most sophisticated computer would be baffled in attempting to analyze the various multilevel claims of the claimants, to identify where they intersect and where they diverge. Therefore, the cells of this diagram are not meant to be filled in in a finite manner. However, it is a useful framework: (1) to illustrate the intricacies of this multivariable situation, (2) to alert us to the dangers of oversimplification in concentrating solely on one factor or one group, (3) to sensitize us to the fact that all these aspects must be acknowledged and understood in negotiating for our rights, and (4) to serve as background for developing models of governance.

Institutional accommodations. Governance models could be thought of as being made up of an additional dimension to be added to this diagram: namely, the structural elements and processes whereby these claims are recognized, negotiated, and satisfied. For these we could return to Barber's classification of accommodative mechanisms within which the professional-institutional dynamic occurs and strains are reduced— differentiated *role* structures, differentiated *authority* structures, and differentiated *reward* structures. Of these, he has explained:

> Organizations that use professionals can usually create for them specialized *roles* in partially segregated substructures of the organization so that the professionals may carry on their own activities as they require. (7:26)

217

(Clinical series or ladders reflecting a hierarchy of nursing expertise and clinical performance illustrate such a role structure.)

> Organizations that use professionals can also usually create a specialized type of *authority* structure which is an accommodation between the organization's need for the pattern of superordinate control and the professional's need for the colleague control pattern of authority. The key role in this accommodative and specialized authority structure is played by the "professional-administrator." The occupant of this role must be a professional who can judge and direct another professional but who can also exercise superordinate control when necessary. (7:27)

(Nurses reporting to nurses is a structural aspect we have long insisted on. Thus a hierarchy of blended clinical-administrative expertise is formed.)

> Organizations that employ professionals can usually create opportunities for them to achieve professional *rewards* while still serving the primary needs of the organization. (7:27)

Examples of professional rewards, beyond financial remuneration, are:

> The opportunity to participate in professional association meetings, to publish research, to continue professional training through tuition subsidies and leaves of absence, to be employed full time on strictly professional work, to be a member of a strong professional group on the job itself, and to advance in salary and prestige for continuing in strictly professional work . . . multiple career channels . . . a "professional ladder." (7:27-28)

(Salary increments, and other benefits commensurate with the hierarchy of clinical and administrative roles, comprise an

---

area of greatest disappointment and most vigorous pursuit in contemporary nursing.)

The critical equation. To the extent that it has control over these structures, the health care institution, with its own vested interest, is in the difficult position of responding to and arbitrating the vested interests (or claims) of the other parties in this interplay. This might even be stated in the form of a governance principle or equation:

> The accommodations of professional-institutional governance should balance the legitimate claims of the claimants.

Or, to fill in the blanks in this set of circumstances:

Governance structures should balance the	*Claims* of the	*Claimants*
Role	Rights	Nurses
Authority	Goals	Patients
Reward	Expertise	Nursing
	Responsibilities	profession
		Other
		professions
		Institutions
		Public

Implications for governance. An equation serves well to identify the ingredients and the relationships in a transaction. However, its seeming precision must not be allowed to mask the untidiness in the actual operation, particularly as relates to complex health care settings. As stated, the equation actually assumes in a sterile sense that a proper balance will prevail, meaning that claims will be settled based on their legitimacy. In practice, however, the claims are negotiated, not granted, and *power* is a key factor in *negotiation*. Therefore, the principle, corrected to reflect the forces and processes of a political environment, would substitute these realities for the idealistic "should":

The *Claims* of the *Claimants* $\xrightarrow{\text{are negotiated}}$
      Rights   Nurses   (POWER as Catalyst)
      Goals   Patients
      Expertise   Nursing
      Responsibilities   profession
                      Other
                      professions
                      Institutions
                      Public

to achieve *Structural Accommodations*
      Role
      Authority
      Reward

Negotiation, meaning to bring about through conference and compromise, occurs at all levels of organization and governance and through formal and informal means. It occurs when the professional association competes with other lobbies in debating reimbursement or nursing practice legislation in Washington, D.C., or the state capital. It occurs when, through collective bargaining or other concerted activities, nursing argues for higher salaries or greater voice in staffing patterns within the institutions. It occurs when the head nurse insists that it would be unsafe and inhumane to add another patient to an already overtaxed unit.

Power, which derives from many sources, including knowledge, is an essential driving force in any accomplishment. It plays a critical role in negotiation and governance. In an untoward sense it may override legitimacy and award one claimant a yield from the role, authority, and reward accommodations out of proportion to the weight of his claims as measured against the claims of others. Thus, it can enable one group to satisfy its claims at the expense of others. Two interrelated sources of power requiring special attention here are the *law*, largely in the form of government regulation of health care agencies and of the professions, and *economics*, as reflected in fee entitlements and granted monopolies.

Physicians possess inordinate leverage in these transactions by virtue of governmental policies relating to reimbursement and health care supervision. They are also in this power seat by virtue of their exclusive rights to bring the client into the system and to dictate his needs/demands for the services of the institution, including that of its other professional employees. Such powers seem to recognize the physician's claims of *expertise* as superseding those of patient's *rights* to self-determination and the *expertise* of others.

As nurses who have long lacked these legal and economic advantages in negotiations, we must recognize their importance and seek changes in these fundamental policies. Also, we must identify and develop strategies to tap other power sources. For example, there is power where our claims overlap those of other claimants and form a basis for forging *coalitions* in the negotiation. Where do our goals merge with those of consumers or other professional groups with respect to needed reimbursement or management reform?

As another example, we should recognize that there is power in *scarcity* of a needed commodity. We stand to gain leverage to force appropriate accommodations during the current situation in which accelerating demand for our expert services is outdistancing the available supply. It is the *responsibility of institutions and government* oversight agencies, wishing to maximize those precious services, to develop and support organizational models that acknowledge nursing's rightful claims along with those of other claimants. It is the *responsibility of the profession and its members* to reinforce those claims in the handling of professional affairs. Drawing on the factors in the equation, this means specifically that, while nursing makes explicit its

rights, goals, expertise, and responsibilities,

successful governance systems, by whatever innovative devices, must reflect these in

role, authority, and reward structures.

Organizational models that overlook one of these key expectations and accommodations are doomed to fail, whereas those that conscientiously strive for balance may well lead to job satisfaction for the nurse and exceptional job performance for her employers and her patients.

Summing up. In this segment on governance models, I have identified a number of factors for consideration. How do they add up to provide guidance in developing an action plan? Essentially, it amounts to this:

Nurses, in designing and developing strategies for achieving governance systems that assure their maximum contribution and return, must recognize and operate according to these understandings:

□ There are *multiple claims* and *claimants* involved.

□ In the *negotiation* process, legitimacy, knowledge, and all other sources of *power* are important and must be identified, established, and utilized.

□ The objectives of the negotiations are
  • role
  • authority, and
  • reward
       accommodations.

□ These accommodations should provide
  • *roles* developed according to the job to be done and the best use of the expertise available

---

222

- appropriate *authority* invested directly within or in support of each role
- *reward* commensurate with the value of the services

□ A *comprehensive approach* to the preceding is essential. Failure to achieve appropriate accommodation within one structure will negate effort with the others.

And thus, the new endowment would swell with those structural elements that form the institutional context for nursing practice and the driving forces to their attainment.

ADDING UP THE NEW ENDOWMENT

It bears repeating that the new endowment refers to the investment of fresh perspective, natural capacity, and power in ourselves—as nurses and as a profession. The details of what each individual and institution contribute to a new nursing endowment remain for our particular creativity and circumstances to determine. However, I believe we should concentrate our efforts in developing and achieving articulation among the general areas of:

Professional models that encompass in an integrated or parallel fashion all necessary facets of the nursing role, ranging from advanced clinical practice to research, to administration, to policy formulation

Academic models that are content driven to their appropriate levels and that mirror the chosen professional models

Socialization models (individuals and programs) that aim for the qualities of social significance, ultimacy of professional performance, and collegiality and collectivity and that embody the interaction elements of identification, instruction, exemplification, appraisal, sanction, collaboration, sponsorship, and institutional acculturation

Governance models that balance the legitimate claims of rights, goals, expertise, and responsibilities of the various claimants, including nurses and nursing, within the role, authority, and reward structures of the health care system

In returning to the concentric diagram of the nursing universe

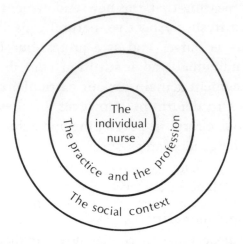

it can be seen that we have created a professional dissonance and a structural disjunction by concentrating our energies on isolated academic systems and professional roles *sans* sufficient scientific content within and contextual support without, somehow assuming these could stand deflated and alone. Previous sections of this book have pointed out the need to enhance the core of the universe through development in the individual of those qualities requisite for professionhood. This final segment on the new endowment emphasizes the importance of the fullness and the fit among the three spheres and the particular attention that must be paid to the institutional and social milieu that surrounds us.

Therefore, coordinated, matched development of these models would constitute capital investments in the future of nursing and would enlarge and strengthen our social contract.

REFERENCE LIST FOR SECTION SIX

1. American Nurses' Association. *A position paper: Educational preparation for nurse practitioners and assistants to nurses.* Kansas City, Missouri: Author, 1965.
2. American Nurses' Association. *Facts about nursing 80-81.* New York: American Journal of Nursing, 1981.
3. American Nurses' Association. Resolutions. *The American Nurse,* 1978, *10*(9), 9-10.
4. American Nurses' Association. Resolutions. *The American Nurse,* 1980, *12*(7), 12-13.
5. Association of Operating Room Nurses, Inc. *Perspectives on entry into practice.* (Adopted by AORN House of Delegates, March, 1979). Denver: Author.
6. Bandler, R., & Grinder, J. *Frogs into princes.* J.O. Stevens (Ed.). Moab, Utah: Real People Press, 1979.
7. Barber, B. Some problems in the sociology of the professions. In K.S. Lynn and the Editors of *Daedalus* (Eds.), *The professions in America.* Boston: Houghton-Mifflin, 1965, pp. 15-34.
8. Brown, E.L. *Nursing for the future.* New York: Russell Sage Foundation, 1948.
9. Cleland, V. The professional model. *American Journal of Nursing,* 1975, 75, 288-292.
10. Dolan, J. Nurses in American history: Three schools—1873. *American Journal of Nursing,* 1975, 75, 989-992.
11. *Facts on File (World News Digest with Index).* June 30, 1978, 38(1964).
12. Grace, H.K. Doctoral education in nursing: Dilemmas and directions. Submitted for publication in 1980 in N.L.Chaska (Ed.), *Views through the mist: The nursing profession* (rev. ed.).
13. Gray, R., & Sauer, K. *Nursing resources and requirements: A guide for state-level planning.* Boulder, Colorado: Western Interstate Commission for Higher Education, 1979.
14. Kramer, M. *Reality shock: Why nurses leave nursing.* St. Louis: The C.V. Mosby Co., 1974.
15. Lieb, I.C. Professional education: Who's in charge? *Chronicle of Higher Education,* 1980, *20*(19), 48.
16. Lysaught, J.P. *An abstract for action.* New York: McGraw-Hill Book Company, 1970.
17. Mauksch, I. Paradox of risk. *AORN Journal,* 1977, *25*(7), 1289-1812.
18. National League for Nursing. *Doctoral programs in nursing 1980-81.* NLN pub. no. 15-1448. New York: Author, 1980.
19. National League for Nursing. *Nursing data book 1979.* NLN pub. no. 19-1797. New York: Author, 1980.

20. National League for Nursing. *State-approved schools of nursing R.N. 1980.* NLN pub. no. 19-1823. New York: Author, 1980.
21. Parsons, T. Professions. In *International encyclopedia of the social sciences* (Vol. 12). New York: Macmillan Co. and The Free Press, 1968, 536ff.
22. Spurr, S.H. *Academic degree structures: Innovative approaches (A general report prepared for the Carnegie Commission on Higher Education).* New York: McGraw-Hill Book Company, 1970.
23. Wandelt, M.A., Hales, G.D., Merwin, C.M., Olsson, N.G., Pierce, P.M., & Widdowson, R.R. *Conditions associated with registered nurse employment in Texas.* Report of Center For Research, School of Nursing, The University of Texas at Austin, 1980.
24. *Webster's New Collegiate Dictionary.* Springfield, Massachusetts: G. & C. Merriam Company, 1973.
25. Western Interstate Commission for Higher Education. *Delphi Survey of Clinical Nursing Research Priorities.* C.A. Lindeman, Principal Investigator. Boulder, Colorado: Author, 1974.

THE VISION

This voiceless dialogue commenced with THE INVITA-TION for you to join me in an uncharted pilgrimage to explore and secure the inner world of nursing. This move was based on the conviction that <u>transformations in nursing begin with transformations</u> within ourselves—in the way we <u>think, feel, and act</u>. Now from a retrospective view, it can be seen that the journey (a year in my time; I hope less in yours) has not followed a streamlined path. As we might expect in proceeding without a roadmap or itinerary, it has suffered false starts, detours, streaks, and bulges. The proof of the joint endeavor lies, though, in whether and how the figure in the mirror has changed.

In this episodic venture, we first stumbled our way through a barren desert on professionalism. Turning from this disappointment to the neglected terrain of ideology, we set our sights on self-actualization and actualization for nursing and scratched out and nurtured a struggling statement of belief about the nature and purpose of nursing. We then paused to examine the meaning of our work in both a personal and impersonal sense, before moving forward reflectively from the ideology to outline the personal qualities needed for us to fulfill our social contract. Finally we burst upon our unexpected destination, looking beyond our own professionhood to the rough foundations of articulated professional, academic, socialization, and governance models as the principal invest-ments for a new nursing endowment.

One final obligation remains.

The essay on *social significance* asserted that this crucial sense is based in large part on a clear conception of nurs-ing—of its social value; of its past, present, and future ac-complishments. In a word, this means VISION, a quality that is a source of inner direction and outward inspiration. The concluding passage on social significance challenged each of us to say specifically what is nursing's actual and potential contribution to society. So I now find myself confronted: Can I? Should I? Will I?

Up to this closing portion, the book has very deliberately followed a reflective vein, attempting to stimulate ways of thinking, to be more provocative than convincing. Specific positions on various issues have appeared only to demonstrate extrapolation from those ways of thinking. On the parting threshold, it seems that I may share the results of my con-templations without abridging yours.

So that which begins with an invitation leads to THE VI-SION, the one I hold for nursing

———

Despite our periodic raillery about the word "nursing" and the perceived stigma attached to this designation, our occu-pation is well named. Nursing is nurturing, nourishing, fos-tering, caring. Nursing is *caring:* both the attitude and the activity. Nursing is caring by promoting health and self-reliance for all. Nursing is caring for those who need to be nurtured in relation to their health status, wherever, as long, and as frequently as they need it, until that need is removed or revised by recovery, independence, or death. This caring responds to needs ranging broadly between the extremes of information and incentive for maintaining wellness to emotional support and technical assistance for sustaining life and providing comfort. As nurses, our MOTIVATION is *caring;* our SERVICES are *caring* and *managing;* our fundamental TOOL is *knowledge,* both tacit and explicit; the PRODUCT of these services is *health*—its maintenance and restoration to the highest possible level of attainment—and physical and psychological *comfort.*

Thus, nursing in its (1) *value dimensions* of holistic health; (2) *geographical dimensions* of home, industry, community, institution; (3) *functional dimensions* of caring and patient and institutional management; and (4) *temporal dimensions* of continuousness, particularly for the institutionalized, is both comprehensive and pivotal. It is comprehensive in that caring in all health states and in all settings is all-encompassing; pivotal in that in primary care, as well as in nursing-intensive institutions, nursing manages or coordinates the variety of caring services around the patient. Nursing *does* encircle the entire clinical (as broadly defined) landscape in health, of which nursing and other professions occupy respective parts, and nursing *should* occupy the total sociopolitical landscape in health, of which others occupy the whole, or nearly so.

NURSING'S UNIQUENESS IS
  less that we hold some exclusive territory and not that
  we are immune from functional redundancy, but
THAT NURSING,
  and nursing alone among the health fields,
IS INCLUSIVE.

231

And patients need inclusivity, perhaps above all else, in our fragmented, mechanistic, superspecialized world.

In the community we are a part of the whole, commingled with environmentalists, public health workers, teachers, social workers, physicians, and so forth. In these settings our particular clinical contribution should be in enhancing health by providing self-care information in understandable, usable forms and in promoting prevention of illness and coping with the stresses of a complex environment; in primary care in clinics; and in home care for the elderly and chronically ill. *In hospitals and nursing homes we surround and penetrate the clinical whole,* in that we both coordinate and provide care. As a wise student once reminded me, "Patients go to hospitals for nursing, not for medical care. If they didn't need nursing, or medical treatments that intensify the need for nursing, they could stay at home."

If we believe in our name and the moral commitment that accompanies it, then we must preserve these broad dimensions; this requires a recommitment to our Nightingale orins. We must not retreat from hospitals and extended care facilities into the community. We must not relinquish technology for sociology and anthropology. We must not abdicate management responsibilities for a narrow individualistic definition of nursing. We must not abandon 24-hour, 365-day nursing for personal convenience and a misguided view of professional prerogative.

On the contrary, we must enlarge our authority in health policy and administration. Where health care is public, we must have a strong hand in governance; where health care is private, we must have a strong hand in ownership—in both instances striving for the best care at reasonable social and personal cost.

Moreover, our clinical hand must be strengthened. New and "expanding" roles, such as those of nurse practitioner and clinical specialist, undoubtedly represent a response to the need for additional nursing knowledge and skills and indicate in a true sense the need for an expanded education, research, and power base for professional practice. Therefore, enlarging and reinforcing our broad dimensions will soon require (1) generic nursing education at the graduate level with a liberal undergraduate base for professional nursing; (2) massive attention to the knowledge base that underlies humanistic and scientific caring within the scope of nursing responsibility; (3) absorption with continuing education to stay abreast of technical advances beyond our wildest dreams and creating enormous pressures on the person and strains within the system; and (4) an international nursing community, bound by mutual interest and respect and instantaneous face-to-face communication capabilities, to maximize our potential and its development.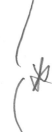

A tide of rising expectations!

- Nursing will become the dominant force in the health care scene.

- Health care will reflect the values of health and human dignity.

- The ideology—that is, belief—will become practice.

- We will clasp hands in solidarity.

- We will say, "I am a nurse" with as much pride and conviction as the Pope and the Queen announce their calling.

Such is my vision, my sense of our social significance.

And the face in the mirror of nursing?

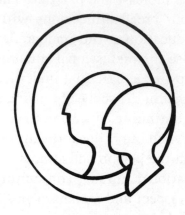

ACKNOWLEDGMENTS

Nancy Evans, in the beginning
  Marilyn Flood, solidly sustaining
    Edith Lewis, above and beyond
      Mary Heatherman
        Jim Grout
          Paul Fitzsimmons
            Sue Kreger
              Tom Brownfield
                Pamela Swearingen, into whose hands

They may know what they have contributed to the work, but never its true value and meaning to the author.

INDEX